THE LOW-FODMAP DIET COOKBOOK FOR FEMALE

Nutritious and Flavorful Meals for Women Managing IBS and Digestive Issues

Sophia Anderson

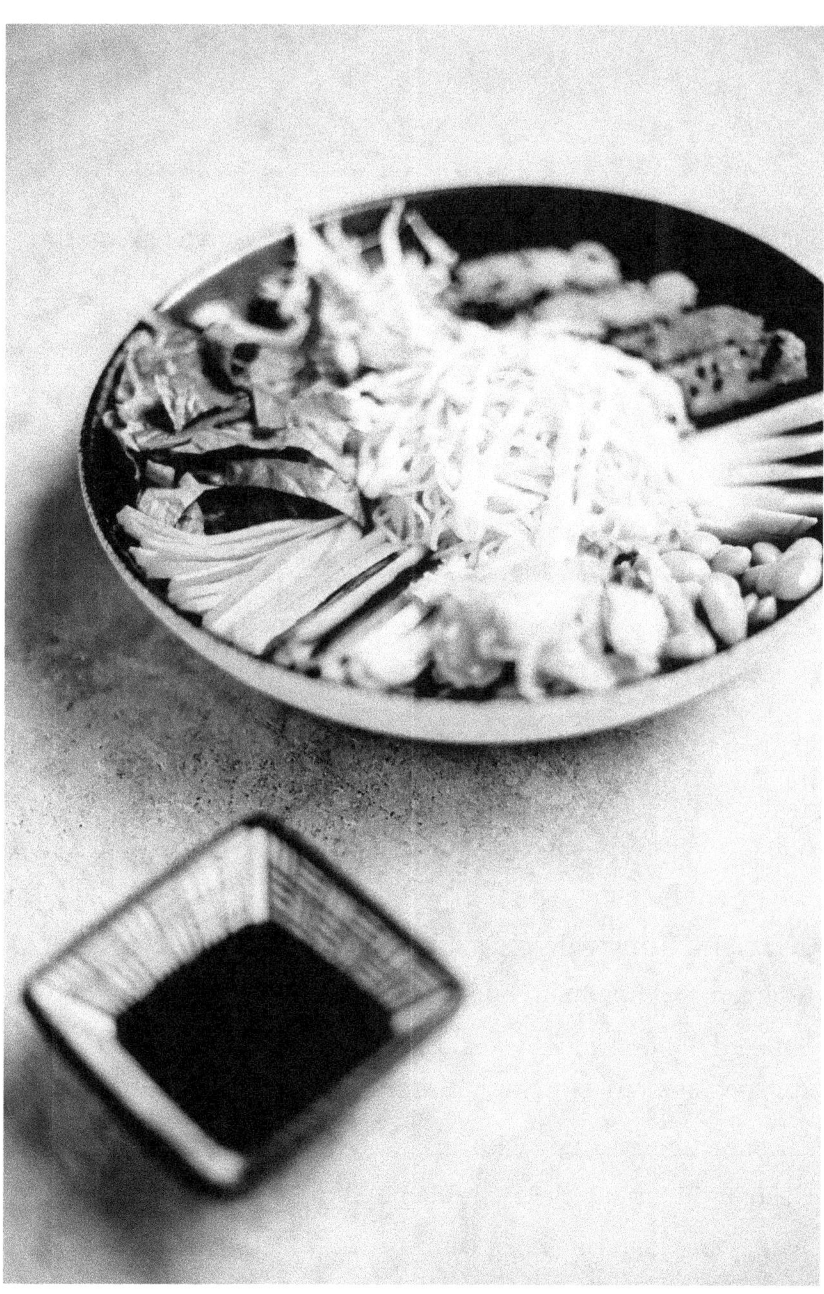

TABLE OF CONTENTS

5

INTRODUCTION

The Low-FODMAP diet has revolutionized the way we approach digestive health, particularly for women. FODMAPs (Fermentable Oligo-, Di-, Mono-saccharides, and Polyols) are types of carbohydrates that can be difficult for some people to digest, leading to a range of uncomfortable symptoms. In this chapter, we will delve into the world of FODMAPs, exploring how they affect digestion and the benefits of the Low-FODMAP diet for women.

FODMAPs: The Hidden Culprits Behind Digestive Discomfort

FODMAPs are found in a wide range of foods, including fruits, vegetables, grains, and dairy products. They are not fully absorbed in the small intestine and instead are fermented by bacteria in the large intestine, producing gas and leading to a range of symptoms.

The main types of FODMAPs are:

- Fructose
- Lactose
- Fructans
- Galactans
- Polyols

The Impact of FODMAPs on Digestion

For women, FODMAPs can have a significant impact on digestive health. The fermentation process can lead to:

- Bloating and gas
- Abdominal pain and cramping
- Diarrhea or constipation
- Nausea and vomiting

Benefits of the Low-FODMAP Diet for Women

The Low-FODMAP diet is a highly effective approach to managing digestive symptoms. By reducing or eliminating FODMAPs from the diet, women can experience:

- Reduced bloating and gas
- Improved abdominal pain and cramping
- Regular bowel movements
- Increased energy and vitality
- Improved overall digestive health

In the following chapters, we will explore the Low-FODMAP diet in more detail, including how to implement it, what foods to avoid and enjoy, and tips for maintaining a healthy and balanced digestive system. By understanding the impact of FODMAPs on digestion and embracing the Low-FODMAP diet, women can take control of their digestive health and enjoy a happier, healthier gut.

Chapter 1: 30 Day Meal Plan

Week 1

Day 1:

- Breakfast: Quinoa Breakfast Bowl

- Lunch: Quinoa Salad with Lemon Herb Dressing

- Dinner: Lemon Herb Baked Salmon

- Snack: Guacamole with Rice Crackers

- Dessert: Chocolate Banana Nice Cream

Day 2:

- Breakfast: Spinach and Tomato Frittata

- Lunch: Chicken and Vegetable Stir-Fry

- Dinner: Turkey and Vegetable Meatloaf

- Snack: Greek Yogurt Dip with Veggies

- Dessert: Almond Flour Brownies

Day 3:

- Breakfast: Banana Oatmeal Pancakes

- Lunch: Turkey and Cranberry Lettuce Wraps

- Dinner: Grilled Steak with Chimichurri Sauce

- Snack: Rice Cake with Almond Butter and Banana

- Dessert: Mixed Berry Crisp with Oat Topping

Day 4:

- Breakfast: Chia Seed Pudding with Berries

- Lunch: Greek Salad with Grilled Chicken

- Dinner: Spaghetti Squash with Marinara Sauce

- Snack: Caprese Skewers with Balsamic Glaze

- Dessert: Lemon Poppy Seed Muffins

Day 5:

- Breakfast: Scrambled Tofu with Vegetables

- Lunch: Tuna Salad Stuffed Avocado

- Dinner: Coconut Curry Chicken with Rice

- Snack: Deviled Eggs with Dill

- Dessert: Coconut Macaroons

Day 6:

- Breakfast: Blueberry Almond Smoothie Bowl

- Lunch: Tomato Basil Soup with Grilled Cheese

- Dinner: Stuffed Bell Peppers with Quinoa and Ground Turkey

- Snack: Trail Mix with Nuts and Seeds

- Dessert: Peanut Butter Energy Balls

Day 7:

- Breakfast: Smoked Salmon and Avocado Toast

- Lunch: Shrimp and Quinoa Spring Rolls

- Dinner: Baked Cod with Roasted Vegetables

- Snack: Hummus and Veggie Platter

- Dessert: Strawberry Shortcake with Coconut Whipped Cream

Week 2

Day 8:

- Breakfast: Greek Yogurt Parfait with Low-FODMAP Granola

- Lunch: Asian Chicken Salad with Sesame Ginger Dressing

- Dinner: Beef and Broccoli Stir-Fry

- Snack: Popcorn with Rosemary and Sea Salt

- Dessert: Chocolate Avocado Pudding

Day 9:

- Breakfast: Zucchini and Feta Egg Muffins

- Lunch: Turkey and Swiss Sandwich on Gluten-Free Bread

- Dinner: Zucchini Noodles with Pesto and Cherry Tomatoes

- Snack: Cucumber Roll-Ups with Cream Cheese and Turkey

- Dessert: Rice Pudding with Cinnamon

Day 10:

- Breakfast: Coconut Flour Waffles with Maple Syrup

- Lunch: Spinach and Strawberry Salad with Balsamic Vinaigrette

- Dinner: Chicken and Vegetable Kabobs

- Snack: Edamame with Sea Salt

- Dessert: Pumpkin Spice Cookies

Day 11:

- Breakfast: Turkey Sausage Breakfast Burrito

- Lunch: Mediterranean Chickpea Salad

- Dinner: Pork Tenderloin with Apple Cider Glaze

- Snack: Rice Crackers with Tuna Salad

- Dessert: Blueberry Lemon Bars

Day 12:

- Breakfast: Overnight Oats with Peanut Butter

- Lunch: Veggie Sushi Rolls with Tamari Sauce

- Dinner: Eggplant Parmesan with Gluten-Free Breadcrumbs

- Snack: Stuffed Mini Peppers with Goat Cheese

- Dessert: Vanilla Bean Panna Cotta

Day 13:

- Breakfast: Veggie Breakfast Casserole

- Lunch: Cauliflower Crust Pizza with Arugula and Prosciutto

- Dinner: Teriyaki Tofu Stir-Fry

- Snack: Sliced Apple with Peanut Butter

- Dessert: Banana Bread with Walnuts

Day 14:

- Breakfast: Green Smoothie with Spinach and Pineapple

- Lunch: Lentil and Vegetable Soup

- Dinner: Moroccan Spiced Chicken with Quinoa Pilaf

- Snack: Turkey and Cheese Roll-Ups

- Dessert: Raspberry Sorbet

Week 3

Day 15:

- Breakfast: Low-FODMAP Breakfast Burrito Bowl

- Lunch: Caprese Salad with Balsamic Glaze

- Dinner: Shrimp and Zucchini Pasta with Lemon Garlic Sauce

- Snack: Veggie Chips with Homemade Salsa

- Dessert: Carrot Cake Cupcakes with Cream Cheese Frosting

Day 16:

- Breakfast: Quinoa Breakfast Bowl

- Lunch: Quinoa Salad with Lemon Herb Dressing

- Dinner: Lemon Herb Baked Salmon

- Snack: Guacamole with Rice Crackers

- Dessert: Chocolate Banana Nice Cream

Day 17:

- Breakfast: Spinach and Tomato Frittata

- Lunch: Chicken and Vegetable Stir-Fry

- Dinner: Turkey and Vegetable Meatloaf

- Snack: Greek Yogurt Dip with Veggies

- Dessert: Almond Flour Brownies

Day 18:

- Breakfast: Banana Oatmeal Pancakes

- Lunch: Turkey and Cranberry Lettuce Wraps

- Dinner: Grilled Steak with Chimichurri Sauce

- Snack: Rice Cake with Almond Butter and Banana

- Dessert: Mixed Berry Crisp with Oat Topping

Day 19:

- Breakfast: Chia Seed Pudding with Berries

- Lunch: Greek Salad with Grilled Chicken

- Dinner: Spaghetti Squash with Marinara Sauce

- Snack: Caprese Skewers with Balsamic Glaze

- Dessert: Lemon Poppy Seed Muffins

Day 20:

- Breakfast: Scrambled Tofu with Vegetables

- Lunch: Tuna Salad Stuffed Avocado

- Dinner: Coconut Curry Chicken with Rice

- Snack: Deviled Eggs with Dill

- Dessert: Coconut Macaroons

Day 21:

- Breakfast: Blueberry Almond Smoothie Bowl

- Lunch: Tomato Basil Soup with Grilled Cheese

- Dinner: Stuffed Bell Peppers with Quinoa and Ground Turkey

- Snack: Trail Mix with Nuts and Seeds

- Dessert: Peanut Butter Energy Balls

Week 4

Day 22:

- Breakfast: Smoked Salmon and Avocado Toast

- Lunch: Shrimp and Quinoa Spring Rolls

- Dinner: Baked Cod with Roasted Vegetables

- Snack: Hummus and Veggie Platter

- Dessert: Strawberry Shortcake with Coconut Whipped Cream

Day 23:

- Breakfast: Greek Yogurt Parfait with Low-FODMAP Granola

- Lunch: Asian Chicken Salad with Sesame Ginger Dressing

- Dinner: Beef and Broccoli Stir-Fry

- Snack: Popcorn with Rosemary and Sea Salt

- Dessert: Chocolate Avocado Pudding

Day 24:

- Breakfast: Zucchini and Feta Egg Muffins

- Lunch: Turkey and Swiss Sandwich on Gluten-Free Bread

- Dinner: Zucchini Noodles with Pesto and Cherry Tomatoes

- Snack: Cucumber Roll-Ups with Cream Cheese and Turkey

- Dessert: Rice Pudding with Cinnamon

Day 25:

- Breakfast: Coconut Flour Waffles with Maple Syrup

- Lunch: Spinach and Strawberry Salad with Balsamic Vinaigrette

- Dinner: Chicken and Vegetable Kabobs

- Snack: Edamame with Sea Salt

- Dessert: Pumpkin Spice Cookies

Day 26:

- Breakfast: Turkey Sausage Breakfast Burrito

- Lunch: Mediterranean Chickpea Salad

- Dinner: Pork Tenderloin with Apple Cider Glaze

- Snack: Rice Crackers with Tuna Salad

- Dessert: Blueberry Lemon Bars

Day 27:

- Breakfast: Overnight Oats with Peanut Butter

- Lunch: Veggie Sushi Rolls with Tamari Sauce

- Dinner: Eggplant Parmesan with Gluten-Free Breadcrumbs

- Snack: Stuffed Mini Peppers with Goat Cheese

- Dessert: Vanilla Bean Panna Cotta

Day 28:

- Breakfast: Veggie Breakfast Casserole

- Lunch: Cauliflower Crust Pizza with Arugula and Prosciutto

- Dinner: Teriyaki Tofu Stir-Fry

- Snack: Sliced Apple with Peanut Butter

- Dessert: Banana Bread with Walnuts

Day 29:

- Breakfast: Green Smoothie with Spinach and Pineapple

- Lunch: Lentil and Vegetable Soup

- Dinner: Moroccan Spiced Chicken with Quinoa Pilaf

- Snack: Turkey and Cheese Roll-Ups

- Dessert: Raspberry Sorbet

Day 30:

- Breakfast: Low-FODMAP Breakfast Burrito Bowl

- Lunch: Caprese Salad with Balsamic Glaze

- Dinner: Shrimp and Zucchini Pasta with Lemon Garlic Sauce

- Snack: Veggie Chips with Homemade Salsa

- Dessert: Carrot Cake Cupcakes with Cream Cheese Frosting

Chapter 2: Breakfast Recipes

This Chapter of our cookbook, where we'll explore delicious breakfast recipes designed to kickstart your day while adhering to a low-FODMAP diet. Each recipe is carefully crafted with flavorful ingredients and easy-to-follow instructions to ensure a satisfying and nourishing morning meal. Let's dive into the recipes and discover new favorites to fuel your mornings!

Quinoa Breakfast Bowl

Ingredients:

- 1/2 cup cooked quinoa

- 1/4 cup sliced strawberries

- 1 tablespoon chopped almonds

- 1 tablespoon maple syrup

- 1/4 teaspoon cinnamon

Instructions:

1. In a bowl, combine cooked quinoa, sliced strawberries, and chopped almonds.

2. Drizzle with maple syrup and sprinkle with cinnamon.

3. Stir gently to combine and enjoy!

Nutrition Information (per serving):

- Calories: 250

- Protein: 6g

- Carbohydrates: 40g

- Fat: 7g

- Fiber: 5g

- Sugar: 10g

- Portion Size: 1 bowl

Spinach and Tomato Frittata

Ingredients:

- 6 eggs

- 1 cup baby spinach leaves

- 1/2 cup cherry tomatoes, halved

- Salt and pepper to taste

- 1 tablespoon olive oil

Instructions:

1. Preheat oven to 350°F (175°C).

2. In a bowl, whisk together eggs, salt, and pepper.

3. Heat olive oil in an oven-safe skillet over medium heat.

4. Add spinach and cherry tomatoes to the skillet and sauté until spinach wilts.

5. Pour egg mixture over the spinach and tomatoes.

6. Cook for 3-4 minutes, then transfer skillet to the oven.

7. Bake for 10-12 minutes or until the frittata is set.

8. Slice and serve hot.

Nutrition Information (per serving):

- Calories: 180

- Protein: 12g

- Carbohydrates: 4g

- Fat: 12g

- Fiber: 1g

- Sugar: 2g

- Portion Size: 1/4 of frittata

Banana Oatmeal Pancakes

Ingredients:

- 1 ripe banana, mashed

- 1/2 cup rolled oats

- 1/4 cup almond milk

- 1 egg

- 1/2 teaspoon vanilla extract

- 1/2 teaspoon cinnamon

- Cooking spray or oil for the pan

Instructions:

1. In a bowl, mix together mashed banana, rolled oats, almond milk, egg, vanilla extract, and cinnamon until well combined.

2. Heat a non-stick skillet or griddle over medium heat and lightly coat with cooking spray or oil.

3. Pour 1/4 cup of the pancake batter onto the skillet and cook until bubbles form on the surface, then flip and cook until golden brown on both sides.

4. Repeat with the remaining batter.

5. Serve hot with your favorite toppings.

Nutrition Information (per serving):

- Calories: 220
- Protein: 8g
- Carbohydrates: 35g
- Fat: 6g
- Fiber: 5g
- Sugar: 10g
- Portion Size: 2 pancakes

Chia Seed Pudding with Berries

Ingredients:

- 1/4 cup chia seeds
- 1 cup almond milk

- 1 tablespoon maple syrup (optional)

- 1/2 cup mixed berries

Instructions:

1. In a jar or bowl, mix together chia seeds, almond milk, and maple syrup (if using).

2. Stir well to combine, then let sit for at least 30 minutes or overnight in the refrigerator to thicken.

3. Once thickened, layer the chia seed pudding with mixed berries in serving glasses or bowls.

4. Serve chilled and enjoy!

Nutrition Information (per serving):

- Calories: 180

- Protein: 5g

- Carbohydrates: 20g

- Fat: 9g

- Fiber: 10g

- Sugar: 5g

- Portion Size: 1 serving

Scrambled Tofu with Vegetables

Ingredients:

- 1/2 block firm tofu, crumbled

- 1/2 bell pepper, diced

- 1/4 cup diced tomatoes

- 1/4 cup spinach leaves

- 1/4 teaspoon turmeric

- Salt and pepper to taste

- 1 tablespoon olive oil

Instructions:

1. Heat olive oil in a skillet over medium heat.

2. Add diced bell pepper and cook until softened, about 3-4 minutes.

3. Add crumbled tofu, diced tomatoes, spinach leaves, turmeric, salt, and pepper to the skillet.

4. Cook, stirring occasionally, until the tofu is heated through and the vegetables are tender, about 5-7 minutes.

5. Serve hot and enjoy!

Nutrition Information (per serving):

- Calories: 150

- Protein: 10g

- Carbohydrates: 8g

- Fat: 9g

- Fiber: 3g

- Sugar: 2g

- Portion Size: 1/2 of recipe

Blueberry Almond Smoothie Bowl

Ingredients:

- 1 frozen banana

- 1/2 cup frozen blueberries

- 1/4 cup almond milk

- 1 tablespoon almond butter

- 1 tablespoon chia seeds

- Toppings of your choice (e.g., sliced almonds, fresh blueberries, granola)

Instructions:

1. In a blender, combine frozen banana, frozen blueberries, almond milk, almond butter, and chia seeds.

2. Blend until smooth and creamy, adding more almond milk if needed to reach desired consistency.

3. Pour the smoothie into a bowl and top with your favorite toppings.

4. Serve immediately and enjoy!

Nutrition Information (per serving):

- Calories: 300

- Protein: 7g

- Carbohydrates: 35g

- Fat: 15g

- Fiber: 9g

- Sugar: 18g

- Portion Size: 1 serving

Smoked Salmon and Avocado Toast

Ingredients:

- 2 slices of low-FODMAP bread, toasted

- 1/2 avocado, mashed

- 2 oz smoked salmon

- 1 tablespoon chopped chives (optional)

- Lemon wedges for serving

Instructions:

1. Spread mashed avocado evenly onto the toasted bread slices.

2. Top each slice with smoked salmon.

3. Sprinkle chopped chives over the smoked salmon, if desired.

4. Serve with lemon wedges on the side for squeezing over the toast.

5. Enjoy your delicious and nutritious smoked salmon and avocado toast!

Nutrition Information (per serving):

- Calories: 250

- Protein: 15g

- Carbohydrates: 15g

- Fat: 15g

- Fiber: 8g

- Sugar: 1g

- Portion Size: 1 serving

Greek Yogurt Parfait with Low-FODMAP Granola

Ingredients:

- 1/2 cup lactose-free Greek yogurt

- 1/4 cup low-FODMAP granola

- 1/4 cup mixed berries (e.g., strawberries, blueberries, raspberries)

- 1 tablespoon honey (optional)

Instructions:

1. In a serving glass or bowl, layer Greek yogurt, low-FODMAP granola, and mixed berries.

2. Repeat the layers until all ingredients are used, ending with a layer of mixed berries on top.

3. Drizzle honey over the top if desired.

4. Serve immediately and enjoy your satisfying and nutritious Greek yogurt parfait!

Nutrition Information (per serving):

- Calories: 250

- Protein: 15g

- Carbohydrates: 30g

- Fat: 8g

- Fiber: 5g

- Sugar: 15g

- Portion Size: 1 serving

Zucchini and Feta Egg Muffins

Ingredients:

- 6 large eggs

- 1 medium zucchini, grated

- 1/4 cup crumbled feta cheese

- 1/4 cup chopped fresh herbs (such as parsley or chives)

- Salt and pepper to taste

- Cooking spray or oil for greasing the muffin tin

Instructions:

1. Preheat your oven to 350°F (175°C) and lightly grease a muffin tin with cooking spray or oil.

2. In a large mixing bowl, whisk together the eggs until well beaten.

3. Stir in the grated zucchini, crumbled feta cheese, chopped herbs, salt, and pepper until evenly combined.

4. Pour the egg mixture evenly into the prepared muffin tin, filling each cup about three-quarters full.

5. Bake in the preheated oven for 20-25 minutes, or until the egg muffins are set and lightly golden on top.

6. Remove from the oven and allow to cool slightly before serving.

7. Enjoy these delicious and nutritious zucchini and feta egg muffins as a satisfying breakfast option!

Nutrition Information (per serving, 2 egg muffins):

- Calories: 180

- Protein: 14g

- Carbohydrates: 4g

- Fat: 12g

- Fiber: 1g

- Sugar: 2g

- Portion Size: 2 egg muffins

Coconut Flour Waffles with Maple Syrup

Ingredients:

- 1/2 cup coconut flour

- 4 eggs

- 1/4 cup almond milk

- 2 tablespoons coconut oil, melted

- 1 tablespoon maple syrup

- 1 teaspoon vanilla extract

- 1/2 teaspoon baking powder

- Pinch of salt

Instructions:

1. Preheat your waffle iron according to manufacturer's instructions.

2. In a large mixing bowl, whisk together the coconut flour, eggs, almond milk, melted coconut oil, maple syrup, vanilla extract, baking powder, and salt until a smooth batter forms.

3. Allow the batter to rest for a few minutes to thicken slightly.

4. Scoop the batter onto the preheated waffle iron, spreading it out evenly, and cook according to manufacturer's instructions until the waffles are golden and crisp.

5. Repeat with the remaining batter.

6. Serve the coconut flour waffles warm with a drizzle of maple syrup and your favorite toppings.

7. Enjoy these fluffy and flavorful coconut flour waffles as a delicious breakfast treat!

Nutrition Information (per serving, 2 waffles):

- Calories: 260

- Protein: 10g

- Carbohydrates: 16g

- Fat: 18g

- Fiber: 8g

- Sugar: 6g

- Portion Size: 2 waffles

Turkey Sausage Breakfast Burrito

Ingredients:

- 2 large eggs

- 2 turkey sausage links, chopped

- 1/4 cup diced bell peppers

- 1/4 cup diced tomatoes

- 2 tablespoons shredded cheddar cheese

- 2 low-FODMAP tortillas

- Salt and pepper to taste

- Cooking spray or oil for cooking

Instructions:

1. In a skillet over medium heat, cook the chopped turkey sausage until browned and cooked through.

2. Add diced bell peppers and diced tomatoes to the skillet and cook until vegetables are tender.

3. In a separate bowl, whisk together the eggs with salt and pepper.

4. Push the sausage and vegetable mixture to one side of the skillet and pour the beaten eggs into the empty side.

5. Scramble the eggs until cooked through, then mix with the sausage and vegetables.

6. Warm the tortillas in the skillet or microwave.

7. Divide the egg mixture between the tortillas, sprinkle with shredded cheddar cheese, and roll up into burritos.

8. Serve hot and enjoy these delicious and satisfying turkey sausage breakfast burritos!

Nutrition Information (per serving):

- Calories: 350

- Protein: 20g

- Carbohydrates: 20g

- Fat: 20g

- Fiber: 3g

- Sugar: 2g

- Portion Size: 1 burrito

Overnight Oats with Peanut Butter

Ingredients:

- 1/2 cup rolled oats

- 1/2 cup lactose-free milk

- 1 tablespoon peanut butter

- 1 tablespoon chia seeds

- 1 tablespoon maple syrup (optional)

- 1/4 teaspoon vanilla extract

- Toppings of your choice (e.g., sliced banana, chopped nuts, berries)

Instructions:

1. In a jar or bowl, combine rolled oats, lactose-free milk, peanut butter, chia seeds, maple syrup (if using), and vanilla extract.

2. Stir well to combine, then cover and refrigerate overnight or for at least 4 hours to allow the oats to soften and absorb the liquid.

3. In the morning, give the overnight oats a stir and add toppings of your choice.

4. Serve chilled and enjoy this convenient and nutritious breakfast option!

Nutrition Information (per serving):
- Calories: 350
- Protein: 10g
- Carbohydrates: 35g
- Fat: 18g
- Fiber: 7g
- Sugar: 8g
- Portion Size: 1 serving

Veggie Breakfast Casserole

Ingredients:
- 6 large eggs
- 1 cup lactose-free milk
- 1 cup diced bell peppers

- 1 cup diced zucchini

- 1 cup diced tomatoes

- 1 cup chopped spinach

- 1/2 cup shredded cheddar cheese

- Salt and pepper to taste

- Cooking spray or oil for greasing the baking dish

Instructions:

1. Preheat your oven to 350°F (175°C) and lightly grease a baking dish with cooking spray or oil.

2. In a large mixing bowl, whisk together the eggs and lactose-free milk until well combined.

3. Stir in the diced bell peppers, zucchini, tomatoes, chopped spinach, shredded cheddar cheese, salt, and pepper.

4. Pour the egg mixture into the prepared baking dish and spread it out evenly.

5. Bake in the preheated oven for 25-30 minutes, or until the casserole is set and the top is golden brown.

6. Remove from the oven and allow to cool slightly before slicing and serving.

7. Enjoy this nutritious and delicious veggie breakfast casserole as a satisfying start to your day!

Nutrition Information (per serving):

- Calories: 200

- Protein: 15g

- Carbohydrates: 10g

- Fat: 12g

- Fiber: 2g

- Sugar: 5g

- Portion Size: 1/6 of casserole

Green Smoothie with Spinach and Pineapple

Ingredients:

- 1 cup spinach leaves

- 1/2 cup frozen pineapple chunks

- 1/2 frozen banana

- 1/2 cup lactose-free milk

- 1/4 cup plain lactose-free yogurt

- 1 tablespoon honey (optional)

Instructions:

1. In a blender, combine spinach leaves, frozen pineapple chunks, frozen banana, lactose-free milk, lactose-free yogurt, and honey (if using).

2. Blend until smooth and creamy, adding more milk if needed to reach desired consistency.

3. Pour into glasses and serve immediately.

4. Enjoy this refreshing and nutrient-packed green smoothie as a healthy breakfast option!

Nutrition Information (per serving):

- Calories: 150

- Protein: 5g

- Carbohydrates: 30g

- Fat: 2g

- Fiber: 4g

- Sugar: 20g

- Portion Size: 1 serving

Low-FODMAP Breakfast Burrito Bowl

Ingredients:

- 1/2 cup cooked quinoa

- 1/4 cup black beans, drained and rinsed

- 1/4 cup diced tomatoes

- 1/4 cup diced bell peppers

- 2 tablespoons sliced black olives

- 1 tablespoon chopped fresh cilantro

- 1 tablespoon lime juice

- Salt and pepper to taste

- Optional toppings: avocado slices, salsa, lactose-free sour cream

Instructions:

1. In a bowl, combine cooked quinoa, black beans, diced tomatoes, diced bell peppers, sliced black olives, chopped fresh cilantro, lime juice, salt, and pepper.

2. Stir well to combine all ingredients.

3. If desired, top with avocado slices, salsa, and lactose-free sour cream.

4. Serve immediately and enjoy this flavorful and nutritious low-FODMAP breakfast burrito bowl!

Nutrition Information (per serving):

- Calories: 250

- Protein: 10g

- Carbohydrates: 40g

- Fat: 5g

- Fiber: 8g

- Sugar: 3g

- Portion Size: 1 serving

Chapter 3: Lunch Recipes

This Chapter of our cookbook, featuring delicious lunch recipes to keep you satisfied and energized throughout your day. Whether you're looking for a quick and easy meal or a more elaborate dish to impress, you'll find something to suit your palate here. Let's dive into these mouthwatering lunch options!

Quinoa Salad with Lemon Herb Dressing

Ingredients:

- 1 cup cooked quinoa

- 1 cup cherry tomatoes, halved

- 1 cucumber, diced

- 1/4 cup red onion, thinly sliced

- 1/4 cup fresh parsley, chopped

- 2 tablespoons olive oil

- 1 tablespoon lemon juice

- 1 teaspoon dried oregano

- Salt and pepper to taste

Instructions:

1. In a large bowl, combine cooked quinoa, cherry tomatoes, cucumber, red onion, and parsley.

2. In a small bowl, whisk together olive oil, lemon juice, dried oregano, salt, and pepper to make the dressing.

3. Pour the dressing over the quinoa salad and toss to combine.

4. Serve chilled or at room temperature.

Nutrition Information:

- Calories: 250

- Protein: 6g

- Carbohydrates: 30g

- Fat: 12g

- Fiber: 5g

- Sugar: 3g

- Portion Size: 1 cup

Chicken and Vegetable Stir-Fry

Ingredients:

- 1 tablespoon olive oil

- 2 boneless, skinless chicken breasts, thinly sliced

- 2 cups mixed vegetables (bell peppers, broccoli, snap peas, carrots)

- 2 cloves garlic, minced

- 2 tablespoons soy sauce (or tamari for gluten-free)

- 1 tablespoon honey

- 1 teaspoon sesame oil

- Cooked rice or quinoa, for serving

Instructions:

1. Heat olive oil in a large skillet over medium heat. Add sliced chicken and cook until browned and cooked through, about 5-6 minutes.

2. Add mixed vegetables and minced garlic to the skillet. Cook until vegetables are tender-crisp, about 4-5 minutes.

3. In a small bowl, whisk together soy sauce, honey, and sesame oil. Pour the sauce over the chicken and vegetables in the skillet.

4. Stir well to coat everything in the sauce. Cook for another 2-3 minutes, until heated through.

5. Serve the chicken and vegetable stir-fry over cooked rice or quinoa.

Nutrition Information:
- Calories: 320
- Protein: 25g
- Carbohydrates: 25g
- Fat: 12g
- Fiber: 4g
- Sugar: 8g
- Portion Size: 1.5 cups

Turkey and Cranberry Lettuce Wraps

Ingredients:

- 1 pound ground turkey

- 1/2 cup dried cranberries

- 1/4 cup sliced almonds

- 2 tablespoons olive oil

- 1 teaspoon ground sage

- Salt and pepper to taste

- Large lettuce leaves, for wrapping

Instructions:

1. In a large skillet, heat olive oil over medium heat. Add ground turkey and cook until browned, breaking it apart with a spoon as it cooks.

2. Stir in dried cranberries, sliced almonds, ground sage, salt, and pepper. Cook for another 2-3 minutes until everything is heated through.

3. Spoon the turkey and cranberry mixture onto large lettuce leaves and wrap them up like a burrito.

4. Serve immediately.

Nutrition Information:

- Calories: 280

- Protein: 22g

- Carbohydrates: 10g

- Fat: 18g

- Fiber: 3g

- Sugar: 5g

- Portion Size: 2 lettuce wraps

Greek Salad with Grilled Chicken

Ingredients:

- 2 boneless, skinless chicken breasts

- 1 tablespoon olive oil

- 1 teaspoon dried oregano

- Salt and pepper to taste

- 4 cups mixed greens

- 1 cup cherry tomatoes, halved

- 1 cucumber, diced

- 1/4 cup Kalamata olives, pitted

- 1/4 cup crumbled feta cheese

- Greek salad dressing, for serving

Instructions:

1. Preheat grill or grill pan to medium-high heat.

2. Rub chicken breasts with olive oil, dried oregano, salt, and pepper.

3. Grill chicken for 6-7 minutes per side, or until cooked through and no longer pink in the center.

4. Let chicken rest for a few minutes, then slice it thinly.

5. In a large bowl, combine mixed greens, cherry tomatoes, cucumber, Kalamata olives, and crumbled feta cheese.

6. Top salad with grilled chicken slices.

7. Drizzle Greek salad dressing over the salad before serving.

Nutrition Information:

- Calories: 320

- Protein: 30g

- Carbohydrates: 10g

- Fat: 18g

- Fiber: 4g

- Sugar: 5g

- Portion Size: 2 cups salad with chicken

Tuna Salad Stuffed Avocado

Ingredients:

- 2 cans (5 oz each) tuna, drained

- 1/4 cup diced red onion

- 1/4 cup diced celery

- 2 tablespoons chopped fresh parsley

- 2 tablespoons mayonnaise

- 1 tablespoon lemon juice

- Salt and pepper to taste

- 2 ripe avocados, halved and pitted

Instructions:

1. In a mixing bowl, combine drained tuna, diced red onion, diced celery, chopped fresh parsley, mayonnaise, and lemon juice. Mix well.

2. Season with salt and pepper to taste.

3. Scoop out some flesh from each avocado half to create a larger cavity.

4. Fill each avocado half with the tuna salad mixture.

5. Serve immediately.

Nutrition Information:

- Calories: 320

- Protein: 20g

- Carbohydrates: 12g

- Fat: 25g

- Fiber: 8g

- Sugar: 2g

- Portion Size: 1 stuffed avocado half

Tomato Basil Soup with Grilled Cheese

Ingredients:

- 1 tablespoon olive oil

- 1 onion, chopped

- 2 cloves garlic, minced

- 4 cups canned diced tomatoes

- 2 cups vegetable broth

- 1/4 cup chopped fresh basil

- Salt and pepper to taste

- 4 slices gluten-free bread

- 1 cup shredded mozzarella cheese

Instructions:

1. Heat olive oil in a large pot over medium heat. Add chopped onion and minced garlic. Cook until onion is soft and translucent, about 5 minutes.

2. Add canned diced tomatoes (with juices) and vegetable broth to the pot. Bring to a simmer and cook for 15-20 minutes.

3. Use an immersion blender to blend the soup until smooth. Alternatively, transfer the soup to a blender and blend until smooth, then return it to the pot.

4. Stir in chopped fresh basil and season with salt and pepper to taste.

5. Meanwhile, preheat a skillet over medium heat. Place two slices of gluten-free bread in the skillet and top each with shredded

mozzarella cheese. Place the remaining bread slices on top to make sandwiches.

6. Cook the sandwiches until the bread is golden brown and the cheese is melted, about 2-3 minutes per side.

7. Serve the tomato basil soup with grilled cheese sandwiches on the side.

Nutrition Information:

- Calories: 380 (soup only)

- Protein: 8g (soup only)

- Carbohydrates: 30g (soup only)

- Fat: 25g (soup only)

- Fiber: 6g (soup only)

- Sugar: 16g (soup only)

- Portion Size: 1 cup soup, 1 grilled cheese sandwich

Shrimp and Quinoa Spring Rolls

Ingredients:

- 12 large shrimp, peeled and deveined

- 1 cup cooked quinoa

- 1 cup shredded carrots

- 1 cup shredded purple cabbage

- 12 rice paper wrappers

- 1/4 cup fresh mint leaves

- 1/4 cup fresh cilantro leaves

- Dipping sauce of choice (such as peanut sauce or sweet chili sauce)

Instructions:

1. Bring a pot of water to a boil. Add the shrimp and cook for 2-3 minutes, until they turn pink and opaque. Remove from water and let cool.

2. Once cooled, slice each shrimp in half lengthwise.

3. Fill a shallow dish with warm water. Dip one rice paper wrapper into the water for about 5-10 seconds until it softens.

4. Place the softened rice paper wrapper on a clean, damp kitchen towel.

5. Arrange a small amount of cooked quinoa, shredded carrots, shredded cabbage, and fresh herbs (mint and cilantro) in the center of the rice paper wrapper.

6. Fold the sides of the wrapper over the filling, then fold the bottom of the wrapper over the filling and roll tightly.

7. Repeat with the remaining ingredients.

8. Serve the shrimp and quinoa spring rolls with your choice of dipping sauce.

Nutrition Information:

- Calories: 90 per spring roll

- Protein: 5g per spring roll

- Carbohydrates: 16g per spring roll

- Fat: 1g per spring roll

- Fiber: 2g per spring roll

- Sugar: 1g per spring roll

- Portion Size: 1 spring roll

Asian Chicken Salad with Sesame Ginger Dressing

Ingredients:

- 2 boneless, skinless chicken breasts

- 6 cups mixed salad greens

- 1 cup shredded red cabbage

- 1 cup shredded carrots

- 1/4 cup sliced almonds

- 2 tablespoons chopped green onions

- Sesame ginger dressing (store-bought or homemade)

Instructions:

1. Season the chicken breasts with salt and pepper. Grill or bake until cooked through, then let cool and slice thinly.

2. In a large bowl, combine mixed salad greens, shredded red cabbage, shredded carrots, sliced almonds, and chopped green onions.

3. Add the sliced chicken to the salad.

4. Drizzle sesame ginger dressing over the salad and toss to combine.

5. Serve immediately.

Nutrition Information:

- Calories: 280

- Protein: 25g

- Carbohydrates: 15g

- Fat: 12g

- Fiber: 5g

- Sugar: 7g

- Portion Size: 2 cups salad with chicken

Turkey and Swiss Sandwich on Gluten-Free Bread

Ingredients:

- 4 slices gluten-free bread

- 8 slices deli turkey

- 4 slices Swiss cheese

- 1/2 cup spinach leaves

- 1/4 cup sliced tomatoes

- Mustard or mayonnaise (optional)

Instructions:

1. If desired, lightly toast the gluten-free bread slices.

2. Layer each slice of bread with 2 slices of deli turkey, 1 slice of Swiss cheese, spinach leaves, and sliced tomatoes.

3. Spread mustard or mayonnaise on one side of the bread slices if desired.

4. Assemble the sandwiches by placing the remaining bread slices on top.

5. Cut the sandwiches in half or enjoy them whole.

Nutrition Information:

- Calories: 320 per sandwich

- Protein: 25g per sandwich

- Carbohydrates: 20g per sandwich

- Fat: 15g per sandwich

- Fiber: 3g per sandwich

- Sugar: 3g per sandwich

- Portion Size: 1 sandwich

Spinach and Strawberry Salad with Balsamic Vinaigrette

Ingredients:

- 6 cups baby spinach leaves

- 1 cup sliced strawberries

- 1/4 cup crumbled feta cheese

- 1/4 cup chopped pecans

- Balsamic vinaigrette dressing (store-bought or homemade)

Instructions:

1. In a large bowl, combine baby spinach leaves, sliced strawberries, crumbled feta cheese, and chopped pecans.

2. Drizzle balsamic vinaigrette dressing over the salad.

3. Toss gently to coat all the ingredients evenly.

4. Serve immediately.

Nutrition Information:

- Calories: 180 per serving

- Protein: 5g per serving

- Carbohydrates: 15g per serving

- Fat: 12g per serving

- Fiber: 4g per serving

- Sugar: 7g per serving

- Portion Size: 2 cups salad

Mediterranean Chickpea Salad

Ingredients:

- 2 cups cooked chickpeas (or canned, drained and rinsed)

- 1 cup diced cucumber

- 1 cup cherry tomatoes, halved

- 1/4 cup diced red onion

- 1/4 cup chopped fresh parsley

- 2 tablespoons extra virgin olive oil

- 1 tablespoon lemon juice

- 1 teaspoon dried oregano

- Salt and pepper to taste

Instructions:

1. In a large bowl, combine cooked chickpeas, diced cucumber, cherry tomatoes, diced red onion, and chopped fresh parsley.

2. In a small bowl, whisk together extra virgin olive oil, lemon juice, dried oregano, salt, and pepper to make the dressing.

3. Pour the dressing over the chickpea salad and toss to combine.

4. Serve chilled or at room temperature.

Nutrition Information:

- Calories: 220

- Protein: 8g

- Carbohydrates: 28g

- Fat: 8g

- Fiber: 8g

- Sugar: 6g

- Portion Size: 1 cup

Veggie Sushi Rolls with Tamari Sauce

Ingredients:

- 4 nori seaweed sheets

- 2 cups cooked sushi rice

- 1/2 cucumber, julienned

- 1/2 avocado, sliced

- 1/2 carrot, julienned

- 1/2 red bell pepper, julienned

- Pickled ginger and wasabi, for serving (optional)

- Tamari sauce or gluten-free soy sauce, for dipping

Instructions:

1. Place a nori seaweed sheet shiny side down on a bamboo sushi mat or a clean kitchen towel.

2. Spread a thin layer of cooked sushi rice evenly over the nori sheet, leaving about 1 inch of space at the top.

3. Arrange julienned cucumber, avocado, carrot, and red bell pepper in a line across the center of the rice.

4. Using the bamboo mat or towel, tightly roll the nori sheet over the filling, pressing gently to seal.

5. Repeat with the remaining nori sheets and filling ingredients.

6. Use a sharp knife to slice each sushi roll into 6-8 pieces.

7. Serve the veggie sushi rolls with pickled ginger, wasabi, and tamari sauce for dipping.

Nutrition Information:

- Calories: 180 per roll

- Protein: 4g per roll

- Carbohydrates: 35g per roll

- Fat: 3g per roll

- Fiber: 5g per roll

- Sugar: 2g per roll

- Portion Size: 1 roll

Cauliflower Crust Pizza with Arugula and Prosciutto

Ingredients:

For the cauliflower crust:

- 1 small head cauliflower, grated

- 1 egg

- 1/4 cup grated Parmesan cheese

- 1/2 teaspoon dried oregano

- 1/2 teaspoon garlic powder

- Salt and pepper to taste

For the toppings:

- 1/2 cup pizza sauce

- 1 cup shredded mozzarella cheese

- 1 cup arugula

- 4 slices prosciutto

- Balsamic glaze for drizzling (optional)

Instructions:

1. Preheat the oven to 425°F (220°C). Line a baking sheet with parchment paper.

2. Place the grated cauliflower in a microwave-safe bowl and microwave on high for 4-5 minutes until softened. Let it cool.

3. Once cooled, transfer the cauliflower to a clean kitchen towel and squeeze out excess moisture.

4. In a large bowl, combine the cauliflower, egg, grated Parmesan cheese, dried oregano, garlic powder, salt, and pepper. Mix well to form a dough.

5. Transfer the cauliflower dough to the prepared baking sheet and press it out into a thin crust, about 1/4 inch thick.

6. Bake the cauliflower crust in the preheated oven for 15-20 minutes until golden brown and crispy around the edges.

7. Remove the crust from the oven and spread pizza sauce evenly over the surface.

8. Sprinkle shredded mozzarella cheese over the sauce, then arrange arugula and prosciutto on top.

9. Return the pizza to the oven and bake for an additional 5-7 minutes until the cheese is melted and bubbly.

10. Remove from the oven and let it cool slightly before slicing.

11. Drizzle with balsamic glaze if desired before serving.

Nutrition Information:

- Calories: 250 per serving (1/4 pizza)

- Protein: 18g per serving

- Carbohydrates: 10g per serving

- Fat: 15g per serving

- Fiber: 3g per serving

- Sugar: 3g per serving

- Portion Size: 1/4 pizza

Lentil and Vegetable Soup

Ingredients:

- 1 tablespoon olive oil

- 1 onion, diced

- 2 carrots, diced

- 2 celery stalks, diced

- 2 cloves garlic, minced

- 1 cup dried green lentils, rinsed

- 6 cups vegetable broth

- 1 bay leaf

- 1 teaspoon dried thyme

- Salt and pepper to taste

- Chopped fresh parsley for garnish (optional)

Instructions:

1. Heat olive oil in a large pot over medium heat. Add diced onion, carrots, and celery. Cook until vegetables are softened, about 5 minutes.

2. Add minced garlic and cook for another minute until fragrant.

3. Stir in dried green lentils, vegetable broth, bay leaf, dried thyme, salt, and pepper.

4. Bring the soup to a boil, then reduce heat and let it simmer for 20-25 minutes until the lentils are tender.

5. Remove the bay leaf and discard.

6. Taste and adjust seasoning if needed.

7. Ladle the lentil and vegetable soup into bowls and garnish with chopped fresh parsley if desired.

8. Serve hot.

Nutrition Information:

- Calories: 220 per serving (1 cup)

- Protein: 12g per serving

- Carbohydrates: 35g per serving

- Fat: 3g per serving

- Fiber: 12g per serving

- Sugar: 6g per serving

- Portion Size: 1 cup

Caprese Salad with Balsamic Glaze

Ingredients:

- 2 large tomatoes, sliced

- 1 ball fresh mozzarella cheese, sliced

- Fresh basil leaves

- Balsamic glaze

- Extra virgin olive oil

- Salt and pepper to taste

Instructions:

1. Arrange the tomato slices and fresh mozzarella slices alternately on a serving platter.

2. Tuck fresh basil leaves between the tomato and mozzarella slices.

3. Drizzle balsamic glaze and extra virgin olive oil over the salad.

4. Season with salt and pepper to taste.

5. Serve immediately as a refreshing and light lunch option.

Nutrition Information:

- Calories: 180 per serving

- Protein: 12g per serving

- Carbohydrates: 8g per serving

- Fat: 12g per serving

- Fiber: 2g per serving

- Sugar: 5g per serving

- Portion Size: 1 plate of salad

Chapter 4: Dinner Recipes

This Chapter of our cookbook, where we dive into delicious dinner recipes to tantalize your taste buds and keep you satisfied. Each recipe is carefully crafted to be both nutritious and flavorful, ensuring that you can enjoy your dinner while adhering to your dietary goals. Let's get cooking!

Lemon Herb Baked Salmon

Ingredients:

- 4 salmon fillets

- 2 tablespoons olive oil

- 2 cloves garlic, minced

- 1 tablespoon lemon juice

- 1 teaspoon dried thyme

- 1 teaspoon dried rosemary

- Salt and pepper to taste

- Lemon slices for garnish

Instructions:

1. Preheat the oven to 375°F (190°C).

2. Place the salmon fillets on a baking sheet lined with parchment paper.

3. In a small bowl, whisk together the olive oil, minced garlic, lemon juice, dried thyme, dried rosemary, salt, and pepper.

4. Pour the herb mixture over the salmon fillets, spreading it evenly.

5. Place lemon slices on top of each fillet for extra flavor.

6. Bake in the preheated oven for 12-15 minutes, or until the salmon is cooked through and flakes easily with a fork.

7. Serve hot and enjoy!

Nutrition Information:

- Calories: 300

- Protein: 25g

- Carbohydrates: 1g

- Fat: 20g

- Fiber: 0g

- Sugar: 0g

- Portion Size: 1 fillet

Turkey and Vegetable Meatloaf

Ingredients:

- 1 lb ground turkey

- 1 onion, finely chopped

- 2 carrots, grated

- 1 zucchini, grated

- 2 cloves garlic, minced

- 1/4 cup ketchup

- 1/4 cup breadcrumbs (gluten-free if desired)

- 1 egg

- 1 teaspoon dried thyme

- 1 teaspoon dried oregano

- Salt and pepper to taste

Instructions:

1. Preheat the oven to 375°F (190°C).

2. In a large bowl, combine the ground turkey, chopped onion, grated carrots, grated zucchini, minced garlic, ketchup, breadcrumbs, egg, dried thyme, dried oregano, salt, and pepper.

3. Mix until well combined.

4. Transfer the mixture to a loaf pan, pressing it down evenly.

5. Bake in the preheated oven for 45-50 minutes, or until the meatloaf is cooked through and golden brown on top.

6. Let it cool for a few minutes before slicing and serving.

7. Enjoy with your favorite sides!

Nutrition Information:

- Calories: 250

- Protein: 20g

- Carbohydrates: 10g

- Fat: 15g

- Fiber: 2g

- Sugar: 4g

- Portion Size: 1 slice

Grilled Steak with Chimichurri Sauce

Ingredients:

- 4 sirloin steaks

- Salt and pepper to taste

- For the Chimichurri Sauce:

  - 1 cup fresh parsley, chopped

  - 1/4 cup fresh cilantro, chopped

  - 3 cloves garlic, minced

  - 1/4 cup red wine vinegar

  - 1/2 cup olive oil

  - 1 tablespoon dried oregano

  - Salt and pepper to taste

  - Red pepper flakes (optional, for heat)

Instructions:

1. Preheat your grill to medium-high heat.

2. Season the steaks with salt and pepper on both sides.

3. Grill the steaks for about 4-5 minutes per side for medium-rare, or until desired doneness is reached.

4. While the steaks are grilling, prepare the chimichurri sauce. In a bowl, combine the chopped parsley, chopped cilantro, minced garlic, red wine vinegar, olive oil, dried oregano, salt, pepper, and red pepper flakes if using. Mix well.

5. Once the steaks are done, remove them from the grill and let them rest for a few minutes.

6. Serve the grilled steaks with a generous drizzle of chimichurri sauce on top.

7. Enjoy your flavorful and juicy steak!

Nutrition Information:

- Calories: 400

- Protein: 30g

- Carbohydrates: 2g

- Fat: 30g

- Fiber: 1g

- Sugar: 0g

- Portion Size: 1 steak

Spaghetti Squash with Marinara Sauce

Ingredients:

- 1 medium spaghetti squash

- 2 cups marinara sauce (store-bought or homemade)

- Fresh basil leaves, for garnish

- Grated Parmesan cheese (optional)

Instructions:

1. Preheat the oven to 400°F (200°C).

2. Cut the spaghetti squash in half lengthwise and scoop out the seeds.

3. Place the squash halves cut side down on a baking sheet lined with parchment paper.

4. Roast in the preheated oven for 40-50 minutes, or until the squash is tender and easily pierced with a fork.

5. Let the squash cool for a few minutes, then use a fork to scrape the flesh into spaghetti-like strands.

6. Heat the marinara sauce in a saucepan over medium heat until warmed through.

7. Serve the spaghetti squash topped with marinara sauce.

8. Garnish with fresh basil leaves and grated Parmesan cheese if desired.

9. Enjoy this light and flavorful dish!

Nutrition Information:

- Calories: 150

- Protein: 2g

- Carbohydrates: 30g

- Fat: 2g

- Fiber: 6g

- Sugar: 12g

- Portion Size: 1 cup of spaghetti squash with marinara sauce

Coconut Curry Chicken with Rice

Ingredients:

- 1 lb chicken breast, cut into bite-sized pieces

- 1 tablespoon coconut oil

- 1 onion, diced

- 2 cloves garlic, minced

- 1 tablespoon curry powder

- 1 can (14 oz) coconut milk

- 1 cup chicken broth

- 2 cups cooked rice (white or brown)

- Salt and pepper to taste

- Fresh cilantro, for garnish

Instructions:

1. Heat the coconut oil in a large skillet over medium heat.

2. Add the diced onion and minced garlic to the skillet and cook until softened, about 2-3 minutes.

3. Add the chicken pieces to the skillet and cook until browned on all sides, about 5-6 minutes.

4. Sprinkle the curry powder over the chicken and stir to coat.

5. Pour in the coconut milk and chicken broth, stirring to combine.

6. Bring the mixture to a simmer and let it cook for 10-15 minutes, or until the chicken is cooked through and the sauce has thickened slightly.

7. Season with salt and pepper to taste.

8. Serve the coconut curry chicken over cooked rice.

9. Garnish with fresh cilantro before serving.

10. Enjoy this aromatic and comforting dish!

Nutrition Information:

- Calories: 400

- Protein: 25g

- Carbohydrates: 30g

- Fat: 20g

- Fiber: 2g

- Sugar: 3g

- Portion Size: 1/4 of the recipe

Stuffed Bell Peppers with Quinoa and Ground Turkey

Ingredients:

- 4 large bell peppers, any color

- 1 lb ground turkey

- 1 onion, diced

- 2 cloves garlic, minced

- 1 cup cooked quinoa

- 1 cup marinara sauce

- 1/2 cup shredded mozzarella cheese

- Salt and pepper to taste

- Fresh parsley, for garnish

Instructions:

1. Preheat the oven to 375°F (190°C).

2. Cut the tops off the bell peppers and remove the seeds and membranes from the inside.

3. In a large skillet, cook the ground turkey over medium heat until browned and cooked through, breaking it up with a spoon as it cooks.

4. Add the diced onion and minced garlic to the skillet with the turkey and cook for an additional 2-3 minutes until softened.

5. Stir in the cooked quinoa and marinara sauce, and season with salt and pepper to taste.

6. Spoon the turkey-quinoa mixture into the hollowed-out bell peppers, dividing it evenly among them.

7. Place the stuffed bell peppers in a baking dish, standing upright.

8. Sprinkle the shredded mozzarella cheese over the tops of the stuffed peppers.

9. Cover the baking dish with foil and bake in the preheated oven for 25-30 minutes.

10. Remove the foil and bake for an additional 5-10 minutes, or until the cheese is melted and bubbly.

11. Garnish with fresh parsley before serving.

12. Enjoy these hearty and nutritious stuffed peppers!

Nutrition Information:

- Calories: 350

- Protein: 25g

- Carbohydrates: 25g

- Fat: 15g

- Fiber: 5g

- Sugar: 8g

- Portion Size: 1 stuffed bell pepper

Baked Cod with Roasted Vegetables

Ingredients:

- 4 cod fillets

- 2 tablespoons olive oil

- 2 cloves garlic, minced

- 1 teaspoon dried thyme

- 1 teaspoon dried rosemary

- Salt and pepper to taste

For the roasted vegetables:

 - 2 cups mixed vegetables (such as bell peppers, zucchini, and cherry tomatoes), chopped

 - 1 tablespoon olive oil

 - Salt and pepper to taste

Instructions:

1. Preheat the oven to 400°F (200°C).

2. Place the cod fillets on a baking sheet lined with parchment paper.

3. In a small bowl, whisk together the olive oil, minced garlic, dried thyme, dried rosemary, salt, and pepper.

4. Pour the herb mixture over the cod fillets, spreading it evenly.

5. In a separate bowl, toss the mixed vegetables with olive oil, salt, and pepper.

6. Arrange the vegetables around the cod fillets on the baking sheet.

7. Bake in the preheated oven for 15-20 minutes, or until the cod is cooked through and flakes easily with a fork.

8. Serve the baked cod with roasted vegetables on the side.

9. Enjoy this simple yet flavorful and nutritious meal!

Nutrition Information:

- Calories: 250

- Protein: 25g

- Carbohydrates: 10g

- Fat: 10g

- Fiber: 3g

- Sugar: 5g

- Portion Size: 1 cod fillet with roasted vegetables

Beef and Broccoli Stir-Fry

Ingredients:

- 1 lb beef sirloin, thinly sliced

- 2 tablespoons soy sauce (or tamari for gluten-free)

- 1 tablespoon oyster sauce

- 1 tablespoon cornstarch

- 2 tablespoons vegetable oil

- 2 cloves garlic, minced

- 1 teaspoon fresh ginger, grated

- 2 cups broccoli florets

- 1 bell pepper, sliced

- Salt and pepper to taste

- Cooked rice, for serving

Instructions:

1. In a bowl, marinate the thinly sliced beef in soy sauce, oyster sauce, and cornstarch. Let it sit for 15-20 minutes.

2. Heat the vegetable oil in a large skillet or wok over high heat.

3. Add the minced garlic and grated ginger to the skillet and cook for 1 minute until fragrant.

4. Add the marinated beef to the skillet and stir-fry for 2-3 minutes until browned.

5. Add the broccoli florets and sliced bell pepper to the skillet and continue to stir-fry for another 3-4 minutes until the vegetables are tender-crisp.

6. Season with salt and pepper to taste.

7. Serve the beef and broccoli stir-fry hot over cooked rice.

8. Enjoy this classic Asian-inspired dish packed with flavor and nutrients!

Nutrition Information:
- Calories: 350
- Protein: 30g
- Carbohydrates: 15g
- Fat: 18g
- Fiber: 4g
- Sugar: 4g
- Portion Size: 1/4 of the recipe

Zucchini Noodles with Pesto and Cherry Tomatoes

Ingredients:

- 4 medium zucchinis

- 1 cup cherry tomatoes, halved

- 1/2 cup basil pesto (store-bought or homemade)

- 2 tablespoons olive oil

- Salt and pepper to taste

- Grated Parmesan cheese, for garnish (optional)

Instructions:

1. Using a spiralizer, spiralize the zucchinis into noodles.

2. Heat the olive oil in a large skillet over medium heat.

3. Add the zucchini noodles to the skillet and sauté for 2-3 minutes until just tender.

4. Add the cherry tomatoes to the skillet and cook for another 1-2 minutes until heated through.

5. Stir in the basil pesto and toss until the zucchini noodles and cherry tomatoes are evenly coated.

6. Season with salt and pepper to taste.

7. Remove from heat and transfer to serving plates.

8. Garnish with grated Parmesan cheese if desired.

9. Enjoy this light and flavorful dish as a nutritious alternative to traditional pasta!

Nutrition Information:

- Calories: 200

- Protein: 5g

- Carbohydrates: 10g

- Fat: 15g

- Fiber: 3g

- Sugar: 5g

- Portion Size: 1/4 of the recipe

Chicken and Vegetable Kabobs

Ingredients:

- 1 lb boneless, skinless chicken breasts, cut into chunks

- 1 red bell pepper, cut into chunks

- 1 yellow bell pepper, cut into chunks

- 1 red onion, cut into chunks

- 1 zucchini, sliced

- 1/4 cup olive oil

- 2 tablespoons lemon juice

- 2 cloves garlic, minced

- 1 teaspoon dried oregano

- Salt and pepper to taste

- Wooden or metal skewers

Instructions:

1. If using wooden skewers, soak them in water for at least 30 minutes to prevent burning.

2. In a bowl, whisk together the olive oil, lemon juice, minced garlic, dried oregano, salt, and pepper to make the marinade.

3. Thread the chicken chunks, bell pepper chunks, red onion chunks, and zucchini slices onto the skewers, alternating between ingredients.

4. Place the skewers in a shallow dish and pour the marinade over them, turning to coat evenly.

5. Cover and refrigerate for at least 30 minutes to marinate.

6. Preheat the grill to medium-high heat.

7. Grill the chicken and vegetable kabobs for 10-12 minutes, turning occasionally, until the chicken is cooked through and the vegetables are tender.

8. Serve hot and enjoy these flavorful and colorful kabobs!

Nutrition Information:

- Calories: 300

- Protein: 25g

- Carbohydrates: 10g

- Fat: 15g

- Fiber: 2g

- Sugar: 5g

Pork Tenderloin with Apple Cider Glaze

Ingredients:

- 1 lb pork tenderloin

- Salt and pepper to taste

- 1 tablespoon olive oil

- 1/2 cup apple cider

- 2 tablespoons honey

- 1 tablespoon Dijon mustard

- 1 teaspoon apple cider vinegar

- 1/2 teaspoon dried thyme

- 1/2 teaspoon cinnamon

- 1/4 teaspoon ground cloves

Instructions:

1. Preheat the oven to 375°F (190°C).

2. Season the pork tenderloin with salt and pepper on all sides.

3. Heat the olive oil in an oven-safe skillet over medium-high heat.

4. Sear the pork tenderloin in the skillet for 2-3 minutes on each side until browned.

5. Transfer the skillet to the preheated oven and roast the pork tenderloin for 20-25 minutes, or until it reaches an internal temperature of 145°F (63°C).

6. While the pork is roasting, prepare the glaze. In a small saucepan, combine the apple cider, honey, Dijon mustard, apple cider vinegar, dried thyme, cinnamon, and ground cloves.

7. Bring the mixture to a simmer over medium heat and let it cook for 5-7 minutes until slightly thickened, stirring occasionally.

8. Once the pork tenderloin is cooked through, remove it from the oven and let it rest for a few minutes.

9. Slice the pork tenderloin and drizzle the apple cider glaze over the slices.

10. Serve hot and enjoy this tender and flavorful dish!

Nutrition Information:

- Calories: 250

- Protein: 25g

- Carbohydrates: 15g

- Fat: 10g

- Fiber: 0g

- Sugar: 12g

- Portion Size: 1/4 of the recipe

Eggplant Parmesan with Gluten-Free Breadcrumbs

Ingredients:

- 1 large eggplant, sliced into rounds

- Salt

- 1 cup gluten-free breadcrumbs

- 1/2 cup grated Parmesan cheese

- 2 eggs, beaten

- 2 cups marinara sauce

- 1 cup shredded mozzarella cheese

- Fresh basil leaves, for garnish

Instructions:

1. Preheat the oven to 375°F (190°C).

2. Place the eggplant slices in a colander and sprinkle them with salt. Let them sit for 20-30 minutes to draw out excess moisture.

3. Rinse the eggplant slices under cold water and pat them dry with paper towels.

4. In a shallow dish, combine the gluten-free breadcrumbs and grated Parmesan cheese.

5. Dip each eggplant slice into the beaten eggs, then dredge them in the breadcrumb mixture, pressing gently to adhere.

6. Place the breaded eggplant slices on a baking sheet lined with parchment paper.

7. Bake in the preheated oven for 20-25 minutes, flipping halfway through, until the eggplant is golden brown and crispy.

8. Spread a thin layer of marinara sauce on the bottom of a baking dish.

9. Arrange the baked eggplant slices in the baking dish, overlapping slightly.

10. Top the eggplant slices with the remaining marinara sauce and shredded mozzarella cheese.

11. Return the baking dish to the oven and bake for an additional 15-20 minutes, or until the cheese is melted and bubbly.

12. Garnish with fresh basil leaves before serving.

13. Enjoy this gluten-free twist on a classic Italian favorite!

Nutrition Information:

- Calories: 300

- Protein: 15g

- Carbohydrates: 25g

- Fat: 15g

- Fiber: 5g

- Sugar: 8g

- Portion Size: 1/4 of the recipe

Teriyaki Tofu Stir-Fry

Ingredients:

- 1 block (14 oz) extra-firm tofu, pressed and cubed

- 2 tablespoons soy sauce (or tamari for gluten-free)

- 2 tablespoons teriyaki sauce

- 1 tablespoon sesame oil

- 2 cloves garlic, minced

- 1 tablespoon fresh ginger, grated

- 2 cups mixed vegetables (such as bell peppers, broccoli, and snap peas), chopped

- Cooked rice or noodles, for serving

- Sesame seeds and sliced green onions, for garnish

Instructions:

1. In a bowl, combine the cubed tofu with soy sauce, teriyaki sauce, sesame oil, minced garlic, and grated ginger. Toss gently to coat the tofu evenly. Let it marinate for at least 15 minutes.

2. Heat a large skillet or wok over medium-high heat. Add the marinated tofu cubes to the skillet, reserving the marinade.

3. Cook the tofu for 5-7 minutes, stirring occasionally, until it is browned and slightly crispy on all sides. Remove the tofu from the skillet and set aside.

4. In the same skillet, add the chopped mixed vegetables and stir-fry for 5-7 minutes until they are tender-crisp.

5. Return the cooked tofu to the skillet with the vegetables, along with the reserved marinade.

6. Cook for an additional 2-3 minutes, stirring constantly, until everything is heated through and well coated in the sauce.

7. Serve the teriyaki tofu stir-fry hot over cooked rice or noodles.

8. Garnish with sesame seeds and sliced green onions before serving.

9. Enjoy this flavorful and satisfying vegetarian stir-fry!

Nutrition Information:

- Calories: 300

- Protein: 15g

- Carbohydrates: 25g

- Fat: 15g

- Fiber: 5g

- Sugar: 8g

- Portion Size: 1/4 of the recipe

Moroccan Spiced Chicken with Quinoa Pilaf

Ingredients:

- 4 boneless, skinless chicken breasts

- 2 tablespoons olive oil

- 2 teaspoons ground cumin

- 1 teaspoon ground coriander

- 1 teaspoon ground paprika

- 1/2 teaspoon ground cinnamon

- Salt and pepper to taste

For the quinoa pilaf:

  - 1 cup quinoa, rinsed

  - 2 cups chicken broth

  - 1/4 cup chopped dried apricots

  - 1/4 cup chopped almonds

  - 2 tablespoons chopped fresh parsley

  - 1 tablespoon lemon juice

Instructions:

1. Preheat the oven to 375°F (190°C).

2. In a small bowl, combine the ground cumin, ground coriander, ground paprika, ground cinnamon, salt, and pepper.

3. Rub the spice mixture over the chicken breasts, coating them evenly.

4. Heat the olive oil in an oven-safe skillet over medium-high heat.

5. Sear the chicken breasts in the skillet for 2-3 minutes on each side until browned.

6. Transfer the skillet to the preheated oven and roast the chicken breasts for 20-25 minutes, or until they are cooked through and no longer pink in the center.

7. While the chicken is roasting, prepare the quinoa pilaf. In a saucepan, bring the chicken broth to a boil.

8. Add the rinsed quinoa to the boiling broth, then reduce the heat to low, cover, and simmer for 15 minutes until the quinoa is cooked and the liquid is absorbed.

9. Fluff the cooked quinoa with a fork, then stir in the chopped dried apricots, chopped almonds, chopped fresh parsley, and lemon juice.

10. Serve the Moroccan spiced chicken hot with quinoa pilaf on the side.

11. Enjoy this aromatic and flavorful dish inspired by Moroccan cuisine!

Nutrition Information:
- Calories: 400
- Protein: 30g
- Carbohydrates: 30g
- Fat: 15g
- Fiber: 5g
- Sugar: 5g
- Portion Size: 1/4 of the recipe

Shrimp and Zucchini Pasta with Lemon Garlic Sauce

Ingredients:
- 8 oz gluten-free pasta (such as spaghetti or fettuccine)
- 1 lb large shrimp, peeled and deveined

- 2 tablespoons olive oil

- 4 cloves garlic, minced

- 2 medium zucchinis, spiralized or thinly sliced

- Zest and juice of 1 lemon

- Salt and pepper to taste

- Fresh parsley, for garnish

- Grated Parmesan cheese (optional)

Instructions:

1. Cook the gluten-free pasta according to the package instructions until al dente. Drain and set aside.

2. In a large skillet, heat the olive oil over medium heat. Add the minced garlic and sauté for 1-2 minutes until fragrant.

3. Add the shrimp to the skillet and cook for 2-3 minutes on each side until pink and opaque.

4. Stir in the spiralized or thinly sliced zucchinis and cook for an additional 2-3 minutes until just tender.

5. Add the cooked pasta to the skillet along with the lemon zest and lemon juice. Toss everything together until well combined.

6. Season with salt and pepper to taste.

7. Remove from heat and garnish with fresh parsley.

8. Serve hot with grated Parmesan cheese if desired.

9. Enjoy this light and refreshing pasta dish bursting with lemon and garlic flavors!

Nutrition Information:

- Calories: 350

- Protein: 25g

- Carbohydrates: 40g

- Fat: 10g

- Fiber: 5g

- Sugar: 5g

- Portion Size: 1/4 of the recipe

Chapter 5: Snacks and Appetizers

This Chapter of our cookbook, where we explore a variety of delicious snacks and appetizers suitable for any occasion. Each recipe is designed with both taste and nutrition in mind, providing you with wholesome options that are easy to prepare and enjoyable to eat. So, let's dive in and discover some delightful snack and appetizer ideas!

Guacamole with Rice Crackers

Ingredients:

- 2 ripe avocados

- 1 small tomato, diced

- 1/4 cup red onion, finely chopped

- 1/4 cup fresh cilantro, chopped

- Juice of 1 lime

- Salt and pepper to taste

- Rice crackers for serving

Instructions:

1. Cut the avocados in half, remove the pits, and scoop the flesh into a bowl.

2. Mash the avocado with a fork until smooth, leaving some chunks for texture.

3. Stir in the diced tomato, chopped red onion, chopped cilantro, lime juice, salt, and pepper.

4. Mix until well combined. Adjust seasoning to taste.

5. Serve the guacamole with rice crackers for dipping.

Nutrition Information (per serving):

- Calories: 150

- Protein: 2g

- Carbohydrates: 9g

- Fat: 13g

- Fiber: 7g

- Sugar: 1g

- Portion Size: 1/4 cup guacamole with 5 rice crackers

Greek Yogurt Dip with Veggies

Ingredients:

- 1 cup Greek yogurt

- 1 tablespoon lemon juice

- 1 teaspoon dried dill

- 1/2 teaspoon garlic powder

- Salt and pepper to taste

- Assorted vegetables for dipping (carrots, cucumbers, bell peppers, etc.)

Instructions:

1. In a bowl, combine the Greek yogurt, lemon juice, dried dill, garlic powder, salt, and pepper.

2. Mix until smooth and well incorporated.

3. Serve the yogurt dip with assorted vegetables for dipping.

Nutrition Information (per serving):

- Calories: 70

- Protein: 8g

- Carbohydrates: 6g

- Fat: 1g

- Fiber: 1g

- Sugar: 4g

- Portion Size: 1/4 cup yogurt dip with assorted vegetables

Rice Cake with Almond Butter and Banana

Ingredients:

- 1 rice cake

- 2 tablespoons almond butter

- 1/2 banana, sliced

Instructions:

1. Spread the almond butter evenly over the rice cake.

2. Top with banana slices.

3. Serve immediately.

Nutrition Information (per serving):

- Calories: 210

- Protein: 5g

- Carbohydrates: 28g

- Fat: 10g

- Fiber: 4g

- Sugar: 8g

- Portion Size: 1 rice cake with toppings

Caprese Skewers with Balsamic Glaze

Ingredients:

- 1 cup cherry tomatoes

- 1 cup fresh mozzarella balls

- 1/4 cup fresh basil leaves

- 2 tablespoons balsamic glaze

Instructions:

1. On small skewers, alternate threading cherry tomatoes, mozzarella balls, and basil leaves.

2. Drizzle with balsamic glaze just before serving.

Nutrition Information (per serving):

- Calories: 110

- Protein: 6g

- Carbohydrates: 6g

- Fat: 7g

- Fiber: 1g

- Sugar: 4g

- Portion Size: 3 skewers

Deviled Eggs with Dill

Ingredients:

- 6 hard-boiled eggs, peeled

- 3 tablespoons mayonnaise

- 1 teaspoon Dijon mustard

- 1 tablespoon fresh dill, chopped

- Salt and pepper to taste

Instructions:

1. Cut the eggs in half lengthwise and remove the yolks.

2. Mash the yolks with mayonnaise, mustard, dill, salt, and pepper.

3. Spoon the yolk mixture back into the egg whites.

4. Garnish with additional dill if desired.

Nutrition Information (per serving):

- Calories: 120

- Protein: 6g

- Carbohydrates: 1g

- Fat: 10g

- Fiber: 0g

- Sugar: 0g

- Portion Size: 2 egg halves

Trail Mix with Nuts and Seeds

Ingredients:

- 1/2 cup almonds

- 1/2 cup walnuts

- 1/4 cup pumpkin seeds

- 1/4 cup sunflower seeds

- 1/4 cup dried cranberries

Instructions:

1. Mix all the ingredients in a bowl.

2. Store in an airtight container until ready to serve.

Nutrition Information (per serving):

- Calories: 200

- Protein: 6g

- Carbohydrates: 12g

- Fat: 16g

- Fiber: 3g

- Sugar: 6g

- Portion Size: 1/4 cup

Hummus and Veggie Platter

Ingredients:

- 1 cup hummus

- Assorted vegetables (carrots, cucumbers, bell peppers, celery)

Instructions:

1. Arrange the hummus in a bowl and place it in the center of a platter.

2. Surround the hummus with assorted vegetables.

Nutrition Information (per serving):

- Calories: 150

- Protein: 4g

- Carbohydrates: 16g

- Fat: 8g

- Fiber: 5g

- Sugar: 4g

- Portion Size: 1/4 cup hummus with vegetables

Popcorn with Rosemary and Sea Salt

Ingredients:

- 1/4 cup popcorn kernels

- 1 tablespoon olive oil

- 1 teaspoon dried rosemary

- Sea salt to taste

Instructions:

1. Heat the olive oil in a large pot over medium heat.

2. Add the popcorn kernels and cover the pot.

3. Shake the pot occasionally until the popping slows down.

4. Remove from heat and sprinkle with rosemary and sea salt.

Nutrition Information (per serving):

- Calories: 120

- Protein: 2g

- Carbohydrates: 14g

- Fat: 6g

- Fiber: 3g

- Sugar: 0g

- Portion Size: 2 cups

Cucumber Roll-Ups with Cream Cheese and Turkey

Ingredients:

- 1 cucumber, sliced lengthwise into thin strips

- 1/4 cup cream cheese

- 4 slices deli turkey

Instructions:

1. Spread cream cheese over each cucumber slice.

2. Place a slice of turkey on top of the cream cheese.

3. Roll up the cucumber slices and secure with a toothpick if needed.

Nutrition Information (per serving):

- Calories: 100

- Protein: 5g

- Carbohydrates: 3g

- Fat: 7g

- Fiber: 1g

- Sugar: 2g

- Portion Size: 4 roll-ups

Edamame with Sea Salt

Ingredients:

- 1 cup edamame (in pods)

- Sea salt to taste

Instructions:

1. Cook the edamame according to package instructions.

2. Sprinkle with sea salt before serving.

Nutrition Information (per serving):

- Calories: 120

- Protein: 11g

- Carbohydrates: 10g

- Fat: 5g

- Fiber: 4g

- Sugar: 2g

- Portion Size: 1 cup

Rice Crackers with Tuna Salad

Ingredients:

- 1 can tuna, drained

- 2 tablespoons mayonnaise

- 1 tablespoon lemon juice

- Salt and pepper to taste

- Rice crackers for serving

Instructions:

1. In a bowl, combine the tuna, mayonnaise, lemon juice, salt, and pepper.

2. Serve the tuna salad on rice crackers.

Nutrition Information (per serving):

- Calories: 150

- Protein: 15g

- Carbohydrates: 5g

- Fat: 8g

- Fiber: 0g

- Sugar: 0g

- Portion Size: 1/4 cup tuna salad with 5 rice crackers

Stuffed Mini Peppers with Goat Cheese

Ingredients:

- 1 cup mini bell peppers

- 1/2 cup goat cheese

- 1 tablespoon fresh herbs (parsley, thyme)

Instructions:

1. Cut the tops off the mini peppers and remove the seeds.

2. Fill each pepper with goat cheese.

3. Sprinkle with fresh herbs.

Nutrition Information (per serving):

- Calories: 80

- Protein: 4g

- Carbohydrates: 6g

- Fat: 5g

- Fiber: 1g

- Sugar: 3g

- Portion Size: 4 stuffed peppers

Sliced Apple with Peanut Butter

Ingredients:

- 1 apple, sliced

- 2 tablespoons peanut butter

Instructions:

1. Slice the apple.

2. Serve with peanut butter for dipping.

Nutrition Information (per serving):

- Calories: 200

- Protein: 4g

- Carbohydrates: 29g

- Fat: 8g

- Fiber: 5g

- Sugar: 18g

- Portion Size: 1 apple with peanut butter

Turkey and Cheese Roll-Ups

Ingredients:

- 4 slices deli turkey

- 4 slices cheese (cheddar, Swiss, or your choice)

- 4 leaves lettuce

Instructions:

1. Lay a slice of cheese on each turkey slice.

2. Place a lettuce leaf on top.

3. Roll up each turkey slice tightly and secure with a toothpick if needed.

Nutrition Information (per serving):

- Calories: 120

- Protein: 10g

- Carbohydrates: 2g

- Fat: 8g

- Fiber: 0g

- Sugar: 1g

- Portion Size: 2 roll-ups

Veggie Chips with Homemade Salsa

Ingredients:

- 1 zucchini, sliced thinly

- 1 sweet potato, sliced thinly

- 1 tablespoon olive oil

- Salt to taste

- 1 cup diced tomatoes

- 1/4 cup red onion, chopped

- 1 tablespoon lime juice

- 1/4 cup cilantro, chopped

- Salt and pepper to taste

Instructions:

1. Preheat the oven to 375°F (190°C).

2. Toss the zucchini and sweet potato slices in olive oil and salt.

3. Arrange in a single layer on a baking sheet and bake for 20-25 minutes, or until crispy.

4. In a bowl, combine the diced tomatoes, red onion, lime juice, cilantro, salt, and pepper to make the salsa.

5. Serve the veggie chips with homemade salsa.

Nutrition Information (per serving):

- Calories: 150

- Protein: 2g

- Carbohydrates: 18g

- Fat: 8g

- Fiber: 3g

- Sugar: 4g

- Portion Size: 1/2 cup veggie chips with 1/4 cup salsa

Chapter 6: Desserts

Welcome to the dessert chapter of our low-FODMAP cookbook! Desserts are often seen as indulgent and sometimes unhealthy, but in this chapter, you will find delicious treats that fit perfectly within a low-FODMAP diet. Let's dive in!

Chocolate Banana Nice Cream

Ingredients:

- 2 ripe bananas, sliced and frozen

- 2 tablespoons unsweetened cocoa powder

- 1 tablespoon almond milk (or any low-FODMAP milk)

- 1 teaspoon vanilla extract

Instructions:

1. Place the frozen banana slices in a food processor.

2. Add cocoa powder, almond milk, and vanilla extract.

3. Blend until smooth and creamy, scraping down the sides as needed.

4. Serve immediately for a soft-serve texture or freeze for 1-2 hours for a firmer consistency.

Nutrition Information (per serving):

- Calories: 105

- Protein: 1g

- Carbohydrates: 27g

- Fat: 1g

- Fiber: 3g

- Sugar: 14g

-Portion Size: Makes 2 servings

Almond Flour Brownies

Ingredients:

- 1 cup almond flour

- 1/2 cup unsweetened cocoa powder

- 1/2 teaspoon baking soda

- 1/4 teaspoon salt

- 3 large eggs

- 1/2 cup coconut oil, melted

- 1/2 cup maple syrup

- 1 teaspoon vanilla extract

Instructions:

1. Preheat the oven to 350°F (175°C). Grease an 8x8-inch baking pan.

2. In a bowl, mix almond flour, cocoa powder, baking soda, and salt.

3. In another bowl, whisk eggs, melted coconut oil, maple syrup, and vanilla extract.

4. Combine wet and dry ingredients until smooth.

5. Pour batter into the prepared pan and spread evenly.

6. Bake for 20-25 minutes or until a toothpick inserted into the centre comes out clean.

7. Let cool completely before cutting into squares.

Nutrition Information (per serving):

- Calories: 210

- Protein: 4g

- Carbohydrates: 16g

- Fat: 16g

- Fiber: 3g

- Sugar: 12g

-Portion Size: Makes 12 brownies

Mixed Berry Crisp with Oat Topping

Ingredients:

- 4 cups mixed berries (blueberries, raspberries, strawberries)

- 1/4 cup maple syrup

- 1 tablespoon lemon juice

- 1 cup rolled oats

- 1/2 cup almond flour

- 1/4 cup coconut oil, melted

- 1/4 cup maple syrup

- 1 teaspoon cinnamon

Instructions:

1. Preheat oven to 350°F (175°C). Grease a baking dish.

2. In a bowl, toss berries with 1/4 cup maple syrup and lemon juice. Spread in the baking dish.

3. In another bowl, combine oats, almond flour, melted coconut oil, 1/4 cup maple syrup, and cinnamon.

4. Spread the oat mixture evenly over the berries.

5. Bake for 30-35 minutes, until the topping is golden and the berries are bubbly.

6. Let cool slightly before serving.

Nutrition Information (per serving):

- Calories: 180

- Protein: 3g

- Carbohydrates: 28g

- Fat: 7g

- Fiber: 5g

- Sugar: 14g

-Portion Size: Makes 6 servings

Lemon Poppy Seed Muffins

Ingredients:

- 1 1/2 cups almond flour

- 1/4 cup coconut flour

- 1/2 teaspoon baking soda

- 1/4 teaspoon salt

- 3 large eggs

- 1/4 cup maple syrup

- 1/4 cup coconut oil, melted

- 1/4 cup lemon juice

- 1 tablespoon lemon zest

- 1 tablespoon poppy seeds

Instructions:

1. Preheat oven to 350°F (175°C). Line a muffin tin with paper liners.

2. In a bowl, mix almond flour, coconut flour, baking soda, and salt.

3. In another bowl, whisk eggs, maple syrup, melted coconut oil, lemon juice, and lemon zest.

4. Combine wet and dry ingredients until smooth, then fold in poppy seeds.

5. Divide batter evenly among muffin cups.

6. Bake for 20-25 minutes or until a toothpick inserted into the center comes out clean.

7. Let cool completely on a wire rack.

Nutrition Information (per serving):

- Calories: 160

- Protein: 5g

- Carbohydrates: 10g

- Fat: 12g

- Fiber: 3g

- Sugar: 7g

-Portion Size: Makes 12 muffins

Coconut Macaroons

Ingredients:

- 3 cups shredded coconut, unsweetened

- 1/2 cup almond flour

- 1/2 cup maple syrup

- 2 large egg whites

- 1 teaspoon vanilla extract

- 1/4 teaspoon salt

Instructions:

1. Preheat oven to 325°F (165°C). Line a baking sheet with parchment paper.

2. In a bowl, combine shredded coconut, almond flour, maple syrup, egg whites, vanilla extract, and salt.

3. Mix until fully combined.

4. Scoop tablespoon-sized portions onto the baking sheet.

5. Bake for 20-25 minutes, until golden brown.

6. Let cool completely on a wire rack.

Nutrition Information (per serving):

- Calories: 140

- Protein: 2g

- Carbohydrates: 10g

- Fat: 11g

- Fiber: 3g

- Sugar: 7g

-Portion Size: Makes 18 macaroons

Peanut Butter Energy Balls

Ingredients:

- 1 cup rolled oats

- 1/2 cup peanut butter (natural, unsweetened)

- 1/4 cup maple syrup

- 1/4 cup almond flour

- 1/4 cup dark chocolate chips (low-FODMAP)

- 1 teaspoon vanilla extract

Instructions:

1. In a bowl, combine all ingredients.

2. Mix well until everything is fully incorporated.

3. Roll into 1-inch balls.

4. Refrigerate for at least 30 minutes before serving.

Nutrition Information (per serving):

- Calories: 110

- Protein: 3g

- Carbohydrates: 11g

- Fat: 6g

- Fiber: 2g

- Sugar: 5g

-Portion Size: Makes 18 energy balls

Strawberry Shortcake with Coconut Whipped Cream

Ingredients:

- 1 1/2 cups almond flour

- 1/4 cup coconut flour

- 1/4 cup coconut oil, melted

- 1/4 cup maple syrup

- 2 large eggs

- 1 teaspoon baking powder

- 1/2 teaspoon baking soda

- 1/4 teaspoon salt

- 1 cup strawberries, sliced

- 1 can coconut milk (refrigerated overnight)

Instructions:

1. Preheat oven to 350°F (175°C). Grease a muffin tin.

2. In a bowl, mix almond flour, coconut flour, baking powder, baking soda, and salt.

3. In another bowl, whisk melted coconut oil, maple syrup, and eggs.

4. Combine wet and dry ingredients until smooth.

5. Divide batter among muffin cups and bake for 15-20 minutes.

6. Let cool completely on a wire rack.

7. For the whipped cream, scoop out the solid part of the chilled coconut milk and whip until fluffy.

8. Slice muffins in half, top with strawberries and coconut whipped cream.

Nutrition Information (per serving):

- Calories: 220

- Protein: 4g

- Carbohydrates: 16g

- Fat: 16g

- Fiber: 4g

- Sugar: 9g

-Portion Size: Makes 6 servings

Chocolate Avocado Pudding

Ingredients:

- 2 ripe avocados

- 1/4 cup unsweetened cocoa powder

- 1/4 cup maple syrup

- 1/4 cup almond milk (or any low-FODMAP milk)

- 1 teaspoon vanilla extract

Instructions:

1. In a blender, combine avocados, cocoa powder, maple syrup, almond milk, and vanilla extract.

2. Blend until smooth and creamy.

3. Refrigerate for at least 30 minutes before serving.

Nutrition Information (per serving):

- Calories: 220

- Protein: 2g

- Carbohydrates: 23g

- Fat: 15g

- Fiber: 7g

- Sugar: 14g

-Portion Size: Makes 4 servings

Rice Pudding with Cinnamon

Ingredients:

- 1 cup cooked white rice

- 2 cups almond milk (or any low-FODMAP milk)

- 1/4 cup maple syrup

- 1 teaspoon vanilla extract

- 1 teaspoon ground cinnamon

- 1 cup cooked white rice

- 2 cups almond milk (or any low-FODMAP milk)

- 1/4 cup maple syrup

- 1 teaspoon vanilla extract

- 1 teaspoon ground cinnamon

Instructions:

1. In a medium saucepan, combine the cooked rice, almond milk, and maple syrup.

2. Cook over medium heat, stirring frequently, until the mixture thickens, about 20 minutes.

3. Stir in vanilla extract and cinnamon.

4. Remove from heat and let cool slightly before serving.

5. Serve warm or chilled, as desired.

Nutrition Information (per serving):

- Calories: 140

- Protein: 2g

- Carbohydrates: 28g

- Fat: 2g

- Fiber: 1g

- Sugar: 12g

-Portion Size: Makes 4 servings

Pumpkin Spice Cookies

Ingredients:

- 1 1/2 cups almond flour

- 1/4 cup coconut flour

- 1/2 cup pumpkin puree

- 1/4 cup maple syrup

- 1/4 cup coconut oil, melted

- 1 teaspoon vanilla extract

- 1 teaspoon ground cinnamon

- 1/2 teaspoon ground nutmeg

- 1/2 teaspoon ground ginger

- 1/4 teaspoon ground cloves

- 1/4 teaspoon salt

- 1/2 teaspoon baking soda

Instructions:

1. Preheat oven to 350°F (175°C). Line a baking sheet with parchment paper.

2. In a bowl, combine almond flour, coconut flour, baking soda, salt, cinnamon, nutmeg, ginger, and cloves.

3. In another bowl, mix pumpkin puree, maple syrup, melted coconut oil, and vanilla extract.

4. Combine wet and dry ingredients until a dough forms.

5. Drop tablespoon-sized portions onto the baking sheet.

6. Flatten slightly and bake for 12-15 minutes, until golden brown.

7. Let cool on the baking sheet for 5 minutes before transferring to a wire rack to cool completely.

Nutrition Information (per serving):
- Calories: 100
- Protein: 2g
- Carbohydrates: 10g
- Fat: 6g
- Fiber: 2g
- Sugar: 5g
-Portion Size: Makes 18 cookies

Blueberry Lemon Bars

Ingredients:

- 1 cup almond flour

- 1/4 cup coconut flour

- 1/4 cup coconut oil, melted

- 1/4 cup maple syrup

- 2 large eggs

- 1/4 cup lemon juice

- 1 tablespoon lemon zest

- 1 cup blueberries

Instructions:

1. Preheat oven to 350°F (175°C). Line an 8x8-inch baking pan with parchment paper.

2. In a bowl, mix almond flour, coconut flour, and coconut oil until crumbly. Press into the bottom of the prepared pan.

3. Bake for 10 minutes or until lightly golden.

4. In another bowl, whisk eggs, maple syrup, lemon juice, and lemon zest.

5. Pour the lemon mixture over the baked crust and sprinkle with blueberries.

6. Bake for an additional 20-25 minutes, until set.

7. Let cool completely before cutting into bars.

Nutrition Information (per serving):

- Calories: 150

- Protein: 3g

- Carbohydrates: 14g

- Fat: 10g

- Fiber: 3g

- Sugar: 8g

-Portion Size:;Makes 12 bars

Vanilla Bean Panna Cotta

Ingredients:

- 2 cups coconut milk

- 1/4 cup maple syrup

- 1 vanilla bean, split and seeds scraped

- 1 tablespoon gelatin

- 3 tablespoons water

Instructions:

1. In a small bowl, sprinkle gelatin over water and let stand for 5 minutes.

2. In a saucepan, combine coconut milk, maple syrup, and vanilla bean seeds. Heat over medium heat until just simmering.

3. Remove from heat and stir in gelatin until completely dissolved.

4. Pour the mixture into ramekins and refrigerate until set, at least 4 hours.

5. Serve chilled.

Nutrition Information (per serving):

- Calories: 170

- Protein: 2g

- Carbohydrates: 15g

- Fat: 12g

- Fiber: 1g

- Sugar: 10g

-Portion Size: Makes 4 servings

Banana Bread with Walnuts

Ingredients:

- 1 1/2 cups almond flour

- 1/2 cup coconut flour

- 3 ripe bananas, mashed

- 1/4 cup maple syrup

- 1/4 cup coconut oil, melted

- 3 large eggs

- 1 teaspoon vanilla extract

- 1 teaspoon baking soda

- 1/2 teaspoon salt

- 1/2 cup chopped walnuts

Instructions:

1. Preheat oven to 350°F (175°C). Grease a loaf pan.

2. In a bowl, mix almond flour, coconut flour, baking soda, and salt.

3. In another bowl, whisk mashed bananas, maple syrup, melted coconut oil, eggs, and vanilla extract.

4. Combine wet and dry ingredients until smooth, then fold in walnuts.

5. Pour batter into the prepared loaf pan and spread evenly.

6. Bake for 45-50 minutes, until a toothpick inserted into the center comes out clean.

7. Let cool completely before slicing.

Nutrition Information (per serving):

- Calories: 210

- Protein: 5g

- Carbohydrates: 20g

- Fat: 13g

- Fiber: 4g

- Sugar: 10g

-Portion Size: Makes 10 slices

Raspberry Sorbet

Ingredients:

- 4 cups fresh raspberries

- 1/2 cup maple syrup

- 1/4 cup lemon juice

- 1 cup water

Instructions:

1. In a blender, combine raspberries, maple syrup, lemon juice, and water.

2. Blend until smooth.

3. Pour the mixture through a fine-mesh strainer to remove seeds.

4. Transfer the strained mixture to an ice cream maker and churn according to the manufacturer's instructions.

5. Transfer to a container and freeze until firm, at least 2 hours.

Nutrition Information (per serving):

- Calories: 80

- Protein: 1g

- Carbohydrates: 20g

- Fat: 0g

- Fiber: 6g

- Sugar: 12g

-Portion Size: Makes 6 servings

Carrot Cake Cupcakes with Cream Cheese Frosting

Ingredients:

- 1 1/2 cups almond flour

- 1/4 cup coconut flour

- 1 teaspoon baking soda

- 1/2 teaspoon salt

- 1 teaspoon ground cinnamon

- 1/4 teaspoon ground nutmeg

- 1/4 teaspoon ground ginger

- 3 large eggs

- 1/2 cup maple syrup

- 1/4 cup coconut oil, melted

- 1 teaspoon vanilla extract

- 1 1/2 cups grated carrots

- 1/2 cup chopped walnuts

Cream Cheese Frosting:

- 8 oz. cream cheese, softened

- 1/4 cup maple syrup

- 1 teaspoon vanilla extract

Instructions:

1. Preheat oven to 350°F (175°C). Line a muffin tin with paper liners.

2. In a bowl, combine almond flour, coconut flour, baking soda, salt, cinnamon, nutmeg, and ginger.

3. In another bowl, whisk eggs, maple syrup, melted coconut oil, and vanilla extract.

4. Combine wet and dry ingredients until smooth, then fold in grated carrots and walnuts.

5. Divide batter evenly among muffin cups.

6. Bake for 20-25 minutes, until a toothpick inserted into the center comes out clean.

7. Let cool completely on a wire rack.

8. For the frosting, beat cream cheese, maple syrup, and vanilla extract until smooth.

9. Frost the cooled cupcakes.

Nutrition Information (per serving):

- Calories: 250

- Protein: 6g

- Carbohydrates: 20g

- Fat: 18g

- Fiber: 4g

- Sugar: 14g

-Portion Size: Makes 12 cupcakes

Chapter 7: Smoothies

Smoothies are a fantastic way to pack a variety of nutrients into a single, delicious meal or snack. They're particularly helpful for those following a low-FODMAP diet, as they can be easily customized to avoid trigger ingredients. Enjoy these smoothies as part of your breakfast routine, a midday snack, or a post-workout refuel.

Berry Blast Smoothie

Ingredients:

- 1 cup strawberries (fresh or frozen)

- 1/2 cup blueberries (fresh or frozen)

- 1/2 cup raspberries (fresh or frozen)

- 1 cup lactose-free almond milk

- 1 tablespoon chia seeds

- 1 teaspoon honey (optional)

Instructions:

1. Combine all ingredients in a blender.

2. Blend until smooth.

3. Pour into a glass and serve immediately.

Nutrition Information:

- Calories: 180

- Protein: 4g

- Carbohydrates: 35g

- Fat: 5g

- Fiber: 8g

- Sugar: 20g

- Portion Size: 1 glass (approximately 12 ounces)

Green Goddess Smoothie

Ingredients:

- 1 cup spinach leaves

- 1/2 avocado

- 1/2 banana

- 1 cup lactose-free coconut water

- 1 tablespoon hemp seeds

- Juice of 1/2 lime

Instructions:

1. Add all ingredients to a blender.

2. Blend until smooth and creamy.

3. Serve immediately.

Nutrition Information:

- Calories: 220

- Protein: 4g

- Carbohydrates: 27g

- Fat: 12g

- Fiber: 8g

- Sugar: 12g

- Portion Size: 1 glass (approximately 12 ounces)

Tropical Turmeric Smoothie

Ingredients:

- 1 cup pineapple chunks (fresh or frozen)

- 1/2 cup mango chunks (fresh or frozen)

- 1 cup lactose-free almond milk

- 1/2 teaspoon ground turmeric

- 1 teaspoon grated fresh ginger

- 1 teaspoon honey (optional)

Instructions:

1. Combine all ingredients in a blender.

2. Blend until smooth.

3. Serve immediately.

Nutrition Information:

- Calories: 200

- Protein: 3g

- Carbohydrates: 45g

- Fat: 3g

- Fiber: 5g

- Sugar: 37g

- Portion Size: 1 glass (approximately 12 ounces)

Peanut Butter Banana Smoothie

Ingredients:

- 1 banana

- 1 tablespoon natural peanut butter

- 1 cup lactose-free almond milk

- 1 tablespoon chia seeds

- 1/2 teaspoon vanilla extract

Instructions:

1. Add all ingredients to a blender.

2. Blend until smooth and creamy.

3. Serve immediately.

Nutrition Information:

- Calories: 280

- Protein: 6g

- Carbohydrates: 40g

- Fat: 12g

- Fiber: 6g

- Sugar: 22g

- Portion Size: 1 glass (approximately 12 ounces)

Chocolate Spinach Smoothie

Ingredients:

- 1 cup spinach leaves

- 1 banana

- 1 tablespoon cocoa powder

- 1 cup lactose-free almond milk

- 1 tablespoon flaxseed meal

Instructions:

1. Place all ingredients in a blender.

2. Blend until smooth.

3. Serve immediately.

Nutrition Information:

- Calories: 230

- Protein: 5g

- Carbohydrates: 40g

- Fat: 7g

- Fiber: 8g

- Sugar: 20g

- Portion Size: 1 glass (approximately 12 ounces)

Mango Coconut Smoothie

Ingredients:

- 1 cup mango chunks (fresh or frozen)

- 1/2 cup coconut yogurt

- 1/2 cup lactose-free coconut milk

- 1 tablespoon shredded coconut

- 1 teaspoon honey (optional)

Instructions:

1. Add all ingredients to a blender.

2. Blend until smooth.

3. Serve immediately.

Nutrition Information:

- Calories: 250

- Protein: 3g

- Carbohydrates: 45g

- Fat: 10g

- Fiber: 4g

- Sugar: 35g

- Portion Size: 1 glass (approximately 12 ounces)

Peach Pie Smoothie

Ingredients:

- 1 cup peach slices (fresh or frozen)

- 1/2 cup lactose-free almond milk

- 1/2 cup lactose-free vanilla yogurt

- 1/2 teaspoon ground cinnamon

- 1 tablespoon oats

Instructions:

1. Combine all ingredients in a blender.

2. Blend until smooth.

3. Serve immediately.

Nutrition Information:

- Calories: 210

- Protein: 5g

- Carbohydrates: 38g

- Fat: 5g

- Fiber: 5g

- Sugar: 22g

- Portion Size: 1 glass (approximately 12 ounces)

Strawberry Pineapple Smoothie

Ingredients:

- 1 cup strawberries (fresh or frozen)

- 1/2 cup pineapple chunks (fresh or frozen)

- 1 cup lactose-free coconut water

- 1 tablespoon chia seeds

Instructions:

1. Add all ingredients to a blender.

2. Blend until smooth.

3. Serve immediately.

Nutrition Information:

- Calories: 180

- Protein: 3g

- Carbohydrates: 40g

- Fat: 2g

- Fiber: 7g

- Sugar: 25g

- Portion Size: 1 glass (approximately 12 ounces)

Cucumber Mint Smoothie

Ingredients:

- 1 cucumber, peeled and chopped

- 1/2 cup fresh mint leaves

- 1/2 avocado

- 1 cup lactose-free coconut water

- Juice of 1/2 lime

Instructions:

1. Place all ingredients in a blender.

2. Blend until smooth.

3. Serve immediately.

Nutrition Information:

- Calories: 150

- Protein: 2g

- Carbohydrates: 14g

- Fat: 10g

- Fiber: 6g

- Sugar: 5g

- Portion Size: 1 glass (approximately 12 ounces)

Blueberry Almond Smoothie

Ingredients:

- 1 cup blueberries (fresh or frozen)

- 1 tablespoon almond butter

- 1 cup lactose-free almond milk

- 1 tablespoon chia seeds

Instructions:

1. Add all ingredients to a blender.

2. Blend until smooth.

3. Serve immediately.

Nutrition Information:

- Calories: 220

- Protein: 4g

- Carbohydrates: 30g

- Fat: 10g

- Fiber: 8g

- Sugar: 20g

- Portion Size: 1 glass (approximately 12 ounces)

Kiwi Kale Smoothie

Ingredients:

- 2 kiwis, peeled and chopped

- 1 cup kale leaves

- 1 banana

- 1 cup lactose-free almond milk

- 1 tablespoon flaxseed meal

Instructions:

1. Combine all ingredients in a blender.

2. Blend until smooth.

3. Serve immediately.

Nutrition Information:

- Calories: 200

- Protein: 4g

- Carbohydrates: 40g

- Fat: 4g

- Fiber: 7g

- Sugar: 25g

- Portion Size: 1 glass (approximately 12 ounces)

Orange Creamsicle Smoothie

Ingredients:

- 1 orange, peeled and segmented

- 1/2 cup lactose-free vanilla yogurt

- 1/2 cup lactose-free almond milk

- 1 tablespoon honey (optional)

- 1/2 teaspoon vanilla extract

Instructions:

1. Add all ingredients to a blender.

2. Blend until smooth.

3. Serve immediately.

Nutrition Information:

- Calories: 190

- Protein: 4g

- Carbohydrates: 35g

- Fat: 3g

- Fiber: 3g

- Sugar: 25g

- Portion Size: 1 glass (approximately 12 ounces)

Raspberry Beet Smoothie

Ingredients:

- 1 cup raspberries (fresh or frozen)

- 1 small cooked beet, chopped

- 1 cup lactose-free almond milk

- 1 tablespoon chia seeds

Instructions:

1. Place all ingredients in a blender.

2. Blend until smooth.

3. Serve immediately.

Nutrition Information:

- Calories: 180

- Protein: 3g

- Carbohydrates: 35g

- Fat: 5g

- Fiber: 8g

- Sugar: 20g

- Portion Size: 1 glass (approximately 12 ounces)

Avocado Lime Smoothie

Ingredients:

- 1/2 avocado

- 1/2 banana

- 1 cup lactose-free almond milk

- Juice of 1 lime

- 1 tablespoon honey (optional)

Instructions:

1. Combine all ingredients in a blender.

2. Blend until smooth.

3. Serve immediately.

Nutrition Information:

- Calories: 210

- Protein: 3g

- Carbohydrates: 29g

- Fat: 11g

- Fiber: 6g

- Sugar: 16g

- Portion Size: 1 glass (approximately 12 ounces)

Pomegranate Berry Smoothie

Ingredients:

- 1/2 cup pomegranate seeds

- 1/2 cup strawberries (fresh or frozen)

- 1/2 cup blueberries (fresh or frozen)

- 1 cup lactose-free almond milk

- 1 tablespoon chia seeds

Instructions:

1. Add all ingredients to a blender.

2. Blend until smooth.

3. Serve immediately.

Nutrition Information:

- Calories: 190

- Protein: 4g

- Carbohydrates: 35g

- Fat: 5g

- Fiber: 7g

- Sugar: 23g

- Portion Size: 1 glass (approximately 12 ounces)

CONCLUSION

Embarking on a low-FODMAP diet is a significant commitment, but for many women, it represents a pathway to better digestive health and improved overall well-being. Throughout this cookbook, we've explored a variety of delicious and nourishing recipes, each designed to align with the principles of the low-FODMAP diet while ensuring that mealtimes remain enjoyable and satisfying.

Reflecting on the Journey

The journey through the low-FODMAP diet can be transformative. By methodically identifying and eliminating high-FODMAP foods, individuals often experience a reduction in symptoms such as bloating, gas, abdominal pain, and other discomforts associated with irritable bowel syndrome (IBS) and similar conditions. This dietary approach is not just about restriction; it's about empowerment and learning to make choices that support a healthier digestive system.

Balancing Nutrition and Enjoyment

One of the key goals in this cookbook was to demonstrate that a low-FODMAP diet doesn't have to be bland or monotonous. The diverse range of recipes provided—from hearty breakfasts to savory dinners, refreshing snacks, and indulgent desserts—proves that you can enjoy a wide variety of flavors and textures while staying within the dietary guidelines.

The ultimate goal is not only to manage symptoms but also to cultivate a sustainable and enjoyable way of eating that enhances your quality of life. By embracing the principles of the low-FODMAP diet, you're taking a proactive step towards better digestive health and overall well-being.

Thank you for allowing this cookbook to be part of your journey. May it serve as a valuable resource and inspiration as you navigate the path to a healthier, happier you.